ESSENTIAL ANTI-INFLAMMATORY RECIPES FOR BEGINNERS

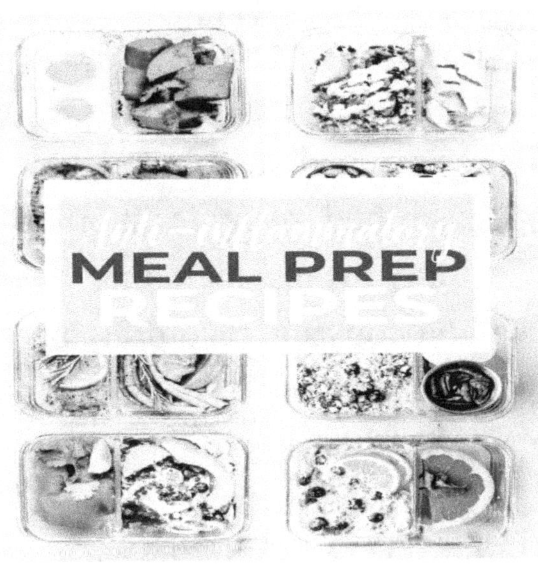

The Beginner's Blueprint to Calm Inflammation and Boost Vitality

PAMELA MONTGOMERY

Copyrighted Material

© 2024 Pamela Montgomery

All rights reserved. No part of this book may be reproduced, distributed, or transmitted in any form or by any means, including photocopying, recording, or other electronic or mechanical methods, without the prior written permission of the publisher, except in the case of brief quotations embodied in critical reviews and certain other noncommercial uses permitted by copyright law.

Copyrighted Material

TABLE OF CONTENTS

Copyrighted Material

Copyrighted Material

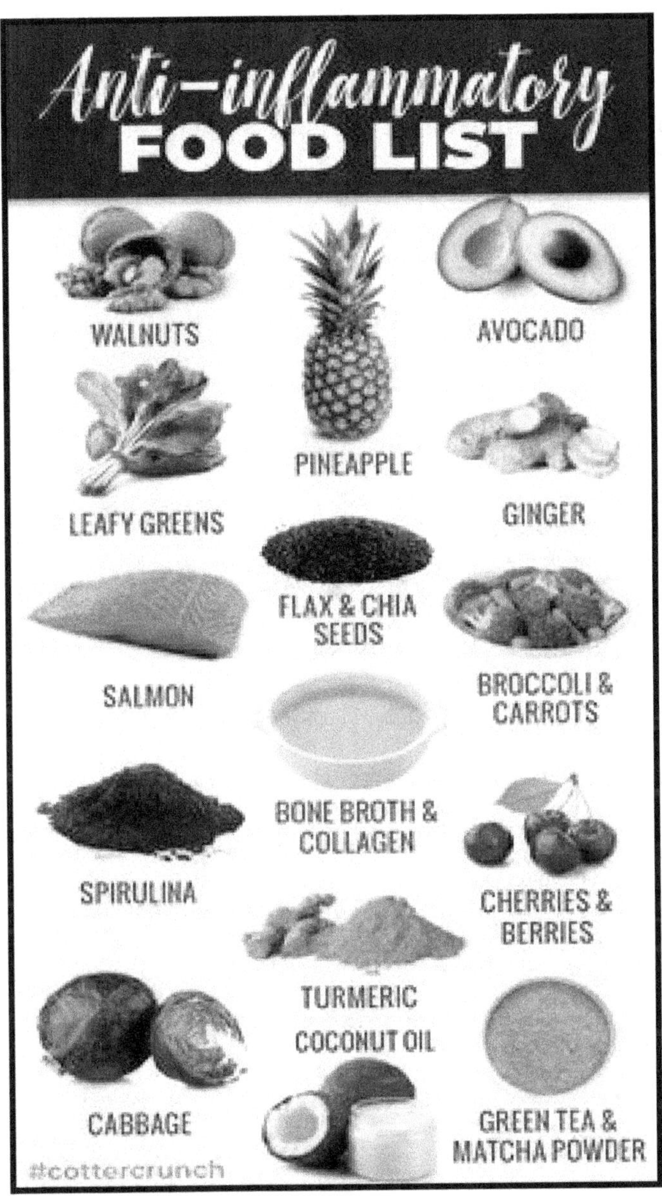

Copyrighted Material

INTRODUCTION

In a world marked by a hectic pace, grasping the intricacies of inflammation is crucial for our well-being. "Essential Anti-Inflammatory Recipes for Beginners" acts as your guide, offering a blueprint for beginners to attain vitality through a calm lifestyle.

Understanding Inflammation

Inflammation, the fiery dance within our tissues. A complicated phenomena that is essential to comprehending our health, it may be a savior or a villain at times. Journeying from the battlefield of acute reaction to the simmering flames of chronic inflammation, let's explore its complexities.

Copyrighted Material

The Body's Defense:

Imagine your body as a bustling fortress. Inflammation is like the sounding alarm when your immune cells detect invaders—be it a rebel splinter, a battalion of bacteria, or even wayward cells. Swiftly, they mobilize, unleashing a torrent of substances like histamine and cytokines. This surge gives rise to the familiar signs: redness, swelling, heat, and pain—the battle flags heralding the onset of the conflict.

Acute vs. Chronic: Knowing the Foe:

- **Acute inflammation:** is the immediate, short-lived response, a precise defense mechanism.
- **Chronic inflammation:** is a lingering fire, is linked to various diseases, arising from autoimmune issues, chronic infections, and lifestyle factors.

Copyrighted Material

Unveiling the Warning Signals:

- **Autoimmune Disorders:** Chronic inflammation can stem from autoimmune diseases, where the immune system mistakenly targets the body's own cells, resembling friendly fire. This internal confusion triggers a prolonged and misguided inflammatory response.

- **Chronic Infections:** The continuous presence of pathogens sustains the inflammatory flames, resembling an unrelenting siege. Chronic infections act as constant provocateurs, keeping the immune system engaged in a prolonged battle.

- **Lifestyle Influences:** Unhealthy dietary choices, chronic stress, and insufficient sleep act as catalysts, intensifying the

Copyrighted Material

inflammatory response. These external factors exacerbate the eternal flame, contributing to the persistence of chronic inflammation.

Building a Fortress of Health: Crafting Your Inflammation-Free Path

Embarking on the journey to an inflammation-free life involves more than just extinguishing the fire; it's about building a resilient fortress. Here's a detailed approach to each crucial element:

Nourish Your Body:

- **Embrace Anti-Inflammatory Foods:** Indulge in a vibrant array of fruits and vegetables, bursting with colors that signify their rich antioxidant and anti-inflammatory properties. Include omega-3-rich fish like salmon or mackerel into your diet, celebrated for their prowess in taming inflammation. These dietary choices fortify your body against inflammatory assaults, supporting overall well-being.

Move Your Body:

- **Exercise as an Anti-Inflammatory Agent:** Physical exercise goes beyond ordinary fitness to become a strong ally against inflammation. Regular exercise, whether via brisk walks, aerobic exercises, or strength training, regulates the inflammatory response, strengthening your body's defensive systems. It is a proactive step toward a life free of inflammation.

Manage Stress:

- **Relax with these Healthy Practices:** Stress, which may cause inflammation, requires a careful approach. Include

Copyrighted Material

stress-reduction practices in your daily routine, such as yoga, meditation, and deep breathing exercises. These techniques not only provide mental peace, but they also contribute to a harmonious internal environment, reducing the inflammatory effect.

Sleep Soundly:

- **The Reparative Power of Sleep**: Prioritize quality sleep as your body's restoration period. During sleep, cells undergo repair, and the immune system strengthens its defenses. Aim for a consistent sleep schedule, ensuring 7-8 hours each night. This rejuvenating rest serves as a cornerstone in fortifying your fortress against inflammation.

By including these components into your daily routine, you build a strong defense mechanism

Copyrighted Material

against the potential dangers of long-term inflammation. Nourishing your body, moving it purposefully, managing stress wisely, and ensuring restful sleep collectively contribute to the construction of your fortress of health, empowering you on your inflammation-free journey.

The Urgency of Addressing Inflammation in Modern Living

Chronic inflammation hides within many of us in today's environment, like a blazing ember hiding under the surface. Though acute inflammation is our body's brave reaction to damage or infection, this low-grade, chronic fire stealthily ravages our health increasing the risk of various diseases.

Copyrighted Material

Why the Urgency?

Modern life bombards us with inflammatory triggers:

- **Processed Foods:** Packed with refined sugars, unhealthy fats, and artificial additives, these increase rapidly the inflammatory response.

- **Stress:** The chronic grind of daily life causes our stress hormones, like cortisol, to remain high, which in turn contributes to inflammation.

- **Lack of Sleep:** Sleep deprivation leads to inflammatory protein production, disrupting the body's balance.

- **Environmental Toxins:** Pollution, pesticides, and chemicals trigger inflammatory responses.

Copyrighted Material

- **Sedentary lifestyle:** Lack of physical exercise weakens our immune system and increases chronic inflammation.

The Oncoming Danger:

This persistent state of inflammation has been related to a multitude of chronic diseases, including:

Heart Disease:

- **Raising Cardiovascular Threats:** Inflammation emerges as a key player in the development of heart diseases, amplifying the risk of heart attacks and strokes. It contributes to the buildup of plaque within the arteries, a key factor in cardiovascular incidents.

Cancer:

- **Fostering Tumor Formation:** Chronic inflammation poses a menace to cellular health, potentially hastening the formation

Copyrighted Material

of cancerous tumors. The inflammatory milieu creates an environment conducive to the initiation and progression of cancer.

Autoimmune Illnesses:

- **Inflammatory Assault on Healthy Cells:** In autoimmune conditions like lupus and rheumatoid arthritis, inflammation drives the immune system to mistakenly target and attack healthy cells. This misguided assault characterizes these persistent conditions.

Brain Disorders:

- **Connecting Chronic Inflammation to Neurodegenerative Ailments:** Chronic inflammation within the brain emerges as a contributing factor to neurodegenerative diseases such as Alzheimer's. The inflammatory response may influence the

Copyrighted Material

advancement of these incapacitating illnesses.

Anxiety and Depression:

- **Impact on Mood and Mental Health:** Beyond its physical consequences, the inflammatory response reaches into mental realms. Anxiety and depression stand out as psychological manifestations intertwined with the systemic effects of chronic inflammation.

Recognizing these intricate connections emphasizes the pivotal need to address and alleviate chronic inflammation for holistic health and well-being. Proactively managing inflammation becomes a cornerstone in preventing a spectrum of illnesses, nurturing a life that is both healthier and more resilient.

Copyrighted Material

Recognizing Early Signs:

Our bodies use minor warning signs to communicate before full-blown illnesses develop. These includes:

Fatigue and Low Energy:

- **Persistent Weariness:** Lingering tiredness and decreased energy levels may serve as initial signs of an underlying health issue.

Unexplained Aches and Pains:

- **Mysterious Discomfort:** Inconsistent or inexplicable aches and pains may serve as the body's whispers, indicating that they should be looked into and attended to.

Difficulty Sleeping:

- **Sleep Disturbances:** Insomnia or disruptions in regular sleep patterns can be indicative of internal shifts affecting overall well-being.

Copyrighted Material

Digestive Issues:

- **Gastrointestinal Discomfort:** Early signs may manifest as digestive disturbances, highlighting potential irregularities in gut health.

Skin Problems like Eczema or Psoriasis:

- **Epidermal Anomalies:** Skin issues such as eczema or psoriasis may surface as external reflections of internal imbalances, urging a closer look at overall health.

Understanding these subtle indicators enables people to take proactive measures to address any health issues before they become worse, highlighting the need for careful self-care and early intervention.

Taking Action: Embracing a Preventative Approach:

Copyrighted Material

Take control and reduce the risks of chronic inflammation with these practical tips:

- **Nourish with Anti-Inflammatory Foods:** Embrace fruits, vegetables, whole grains, and healthy fats.
- **Regular Exercise:** Reduces inflammation and strengthens the immune system. Aim for at least 30 minutes of moderate-intensity exercise most days of the week.
- **Stress Management:** Find healthy strategies to deal with stress, such as meditation, yoga, or spending time outside.
- **Prioritize Sleep:** Aim for 7-8 hours of quality sleep nightly.
- **Minimize Toxin Exposure:** Choose organic foods, filter water, and avoid harsh chemicals.

Copyrighted Material

- **Support Gut Health:** Consume fermented foods, and probiotics, and limit processed foods.

Addressing inflammation isn't just about short-term relief; it's an investment in long-term health. Small lifestyle changes and awareness of modern triggers can help put an end to the inflammation within, promoting a vibrant and resilient life.

Importance of Anti-Inflammatory Diets

In the battle against chronic inflammation, our plates become powerful arsenals, holding the key to a healthier life. An anti-inflammatory diet, armed with the right nutrients, can be your secret weapon in this fight. Let's explore the

Copyrighted Material

importance of embracing the power of food to quell the inflammatory fire within.

Why Go on an Anti-Inflammatory Diet?

Chronic inflammation, a hidden threat, is linked to various modern diseases, from heart disease and cancer to autoimmune disorders and depression. It acts like a slow-burning fire, damaging tissues over time. The good news is that our plates can play a crucial role. An anti-inflammatory diet, rich in nutrients, acts as a shield, protecting cells and reducing inflammation.

Nature's Anti-Inflammatory Arsenal:

Anti-inflammatory foods act as a superfood squad, each with a unique punch against inflammation:

- **Fruits and Vegetables:** These vibrant warriors are Loaded with antioxidants and anti-inflammatory compounds, including

Copyrighted Material

beta-carotene and quercetin. Think berries, leafy greens, bell peppers, tomatoes, and cruciferous vegetables like broccoli and kale.

- **Fatty Fish:** Salmon, tuna, sardines, and mackerel are high in omega-3 fatty acids, which are powerful anti-inflammatory agents that decrease the synthesis of inflammatory molecules.

- **Nuts and Seeds:** Almonds, walnuts, chia seeds, and flaxseeds are high in fiber, vitamin E, and omega-3 fatty acids, making them powerful anti-inflammatory foods.

- **Whole Grains:** Choose brown rice, quinoa, and oats over processed grains. These complex carbohydrates give continuous energy while reducing inflammation.

Copyrighted Material

- **Herbs and Spices:** Turmeric, ginger, garlic, and rosemary are flavorful and potent anti-inflammatory powerhouses.

Building Your Anti-Inflammatory Plate:

Now, let's turn these superfoods into a vibrant feast! Here are practical tips for building an anti-inflammatory plate:

Vibrant Fruits and Vegetables:

- **Boost Nutrient Intake:** Fill half your plate with a variety of colorful fruits and vegetables to ensure a rich mix of nutrients that combat inflammation.

Balanced Protein Sources:

- **Foundation for Balanced Meals:** Include a healthy protein source in every meal, such as fatty fish, poultry, beans, or lentils. These options provide essential nutrients for overall well-being.

Copyrighted Material

Whole Grains for Sustained Energy:

- **Feel Full and Energized:** Opt for whole grains like brown rice, quinoa, and oats instead of refined grains. These choices provide lasting energy, preventing inflammation.

Healthy Fats for Cellular Nourishment:

- **Support Cell Health:** Drizzle olive oil on your salad or snack on nuts and seeds to include healthy fats. These choices contribute to cellular health and overall vitality.

Spices for Flavor and Wellness:

- **Add a Flavorful Kick:** Infuse your meals with turmeric, ginger, and garlic for both enhanced flavor and a potent anti-inflammatory boost.

Copyrighted Material

Hydration for Optimal Functioning:

- **Essential Toxin Flush:** Stay hydrated with water to flush out toxins and support optimal bodily functions. Sufficient hydration is fundamental to an inflammation-free lifestyle.

Incorporating these elements into your meals not only creates a delightful culinary experience but also actively supports your body in the ongoing battle against inflammation.

Beyond the Plate:

While food is a potent weapon in the battle against inflammation, it's just one aspect of the broader puzzle. Remember to complement your anti-inflammatory diet with additional healthy lifestyle practices such as regular exercise, effective stress management, and ensuring adequate sleep. By combining these tools, you create a comprehensive shield against chronic

Copyrighted Material

inflammation, paving the way for a healthier and more vibrant life.

So, take charge of your health, harness the strength of an anti-inflammatory diet, and shift the balance against the silent fire within. You've got the power!

Whether you're new to the realm of anti-inflammatory living or seeking a comprehensive guide to reinforce your knowledge, **"Essential Anti-Inflammatory Recipes for Beginners"** stands as your essential resource for embracing a lifestyle that prioritizes holistic wellness and vitality.

Copyrighted Material

CHAPTER 1: THE BASICS OF ANTI-INFLAMMATORY EATING

Key Principles

Welcome to the heart of anti-inflammatory eating, where I reveal the core principles laying the foundation for a healthier, inflammation-free lifestyle.

Embarking on an anti-inflammatory journey begins with a mindful approach to food choices. Adopting a diet abundant in nutrients and celebrated for its anti-inflammatory properties can significantly impact overall well-being. Let's explore the key principles guiding this transformative lifestyle:

Copyrighted Material

- **Nutrient-Rich Choices:** Choose whole, nutrient-dense foods that fuel the body and counter inflammation. Embrace a vibrant array of fruits, vegetables, lean proteins, and whole grains.

- **Anti-Inflammatory Superstars:** Integrate specific foods renowned for their anti-inflammatory prowess. Include fatty fish like salmon, rich in omega-3 fatty acids, and infuse spices such as turmeric and ginger into your culinary repertoire.

- **Balancing Omega-3 and Omega-6 Fatty Acids:** Aim for an omega-3 to omega-6 fatty acid ratio that is balanced. While omega-6 is essential, an imbalance can contribute to inflammation. Sources of omega-3 include fish, chia seeds, and flaxseeds.

Copyrighted Material

- **Mindful Cooking Techniques:** Choose cooking methods that maintain the nutritional value of foods. Experiment with steaming, sautéing, or baking to retain the goodness in your meals.

- **Limiting Processed Foods:** Minimize processed and refined foods known for their inflammatory potential. Instead, focus on whole, unprocessed options to support your body's natural defenses.

- **Hydration as a Cornerstone:** Prioritize hydration with water and herbal teas. Staying well-hydrated supports bodily functions and aids in flushing out toxins.

- **Gut Health Optimization:** Cultivate a healthy gut microbiome by incorporating probiotic-rich foods like yogurt, kefir, and fermented vegetables. Prebiotic foods

Copyrighted Material

such as garlic and onions further support beneficial bacteria.

- **Moderation and Individualization:** Embrace a balanced approach to eating, recognizing that individual responses to foods may vary. Moderation is key to enjoying a variety of foods without overwhelming the system.

- **Mindful Eating Practices:** Try to develop mindful eating habits by savoring each bite, chewing thoroughly, and being attuned to hunger and fullness cues. Mindful eating fosters a deeper connection with the nutritional experience.

- **Strategic Meal Planning:** Plan meals thoughtfully, ensuring a diverse and well-rounded intake of nutrients. This approach simplifies grocery shopping and

Copyrighted Material

encourages a consistent commitment to anti-inflammatory choices.

- **Incorporating Anti-Inflammatory Herbs:** Explore the benefits of herbs like basil, rosemary, and oregano, known for their anti-inflammatory properties. Infuse these herbs into your dishes for both flavor and health.

- **Stress Management Integration:** Acknowledge the connection between stress and inflammation. Incorporate stress-reducing practices such as meditation, deep breathing, or regular physical activity to complement your dietary efforts.

Remember, the journey to an inflammation-free lifestyle is an ongoing process. By embracing these principles and tailoring them to your

Copyrighted Material

preferences, you pave the way for sustained well-being and vitality.

Building Your Anti-Inflammatory Plate

Imagine a plate bursting with vivid colors, diverse textures, and enticing aromas. This isn't just a culinary masterpiece; it's a formidable defense against chronic inflammation, the stealthy adversary hidden within our bodies. Linked to a range of health issues, from heart disease to autoimmune disorders, chronic inflammation poses a significant threat. The exciting news is, we can combat it not with pills, but with the powerful choices on our plates!

Copyrighted Material

How do you create a plate that's both delectable and health-promoting? Here are the key principles:

- **Plant Power:** Load up on veggies! Aim for half your plate to be a rainbow of non-starchy vegetables. Broccoli, bell peppers, leafy greens, tomatoes – packed with antioxidants and phytonutrients that combat inflammation.

- **Lean and Green:** Opt for lean proteins like grilled chicken, salmon, or tofu for a quarter of your plate. Essential nutrients without excess saturated fat.

- **Whole Grains Rule:** Skip the white choices; embrace whole grains like quinoa or brown rice for the remaining quarter. Complex carbs and fiber keep you energized and satisfied.

Copyrighted Material

- **Healthy Fat Fiesta:** Drizzle olive oil, sprinkle nuts or seeds, or add avocado for your healthy fats. Beyond flavor, they bring anti-inflammatory properties to the table.

- **Spice Up Your Life:** Turmeric, ginger, garlic, and chili peppers – more than just flavors; they fight inflammation. Don't shy away from these culinary warriors!

- **Hydration Hero:** Water is essential! To help you eliminate toxins, try to drink eight glasses a day. Herbal teas and infused waters add flavor to your hydration routine.

- **Mindful Moderation:** Indulge occasionally, but skip sugary desserts, processed snacks, and excess red meat. They can incite inflammation and hinder your anti-inflammatory efforts.

Copyrighted Material

- **Get Creative:** Consider this a template. Experiment with different flavors, textures, and cooking methods to keep your meals exciting and delicious.

- **Make it a Lifestyle:** Anti-inflammatory eating is a lasting commitment. Integrate these principles into your daily routine for a thriving well-being.

- **Celebrate the Journey:** Relish the process of preparing and sharing nourishing meals. Turn on music, light candles, and create a mindful, enjoyable dining experience.

Remember, crafting an anti-inflammatory plate invests in your future health and happiness. With every bite, you're not just pleasing your taste buds but nurturing your body to combat inflammation and flourish. So, get cooking,

Copyrighted Material

explore, and relish your anti-inflammatory culinary journey!

The Links Between Chronic Inflammation and Health Issues

Chronic inflammation, unlike the swift response to a scraped knee, silently smolders within the body. It's a persistent, low-grade immune reaction that, over time, can contribute to a range of chronic diseases. Picture it as a microscopic army on constant high alert, attacking not only invaders but also healthy tissues.

Understanding the Link:

Chronic inflammation can be triggered by various factors, including:

- **Diet:** Excessive sugar, processed foods, and unhealthy fats can fuel inflammation.

Copyrighted Material

- **Stress:** Prolonged stress can release hormones triggering inflammation.

- **Autoimmune diseases:** In these conditions, the immune system mistakenly attacks the body's tissues, leading to chronic inflammation.

- **Infections:** Some chronic infections, like hepatitis, can result in ongoing inflammation.

- **Smoking and pollution:** These can harm tissues and provoke inflammatory responses.

The Health Risks:

This ongoing inflammation can disrupt various bodily systems, putting you at an increased risk for:

- **Heart disease:** Inflammation damages blood vessels, contributing to plaque

Copyrighted Material

buildup and increasing the risk of heart attacks and strokes.

- **Cancer:** Chronic inflammation fosters an environment conducive to cancer cell growth.

- **Autoimmune diseases:** Conditions like rheumatoid arthritis and lupus involve chronic inflammation attacking healthy tissues.

- **Type 2 diabetes:** Inflammation can impair the body's insulin use, leading to high blood sugar levels.

- **Neurodegenerative diseases:** Chronic inflammation is linked to an increased risk of Alzheimer's disease and Parkinson's disease.

- **Depression and anxiety:** Inflammation may play a role in the development of mental health conditions.

Copyrighted Material

Breaking the Cycle: Taking Control of Chronic Inflammation

The good news is that, despite its potency, we have the means to fight back! By adopting an anti-inflammatory lifestyle, we can reduce inflammation and mitigate its harmful effects. Here are the key steps:

- **Embrace an anti-inflammatory diet:** Prioritize fruits, vegetables, whole grains, and lean protein while limiting processed foods, sugary drinks, and unhealthy fats.

- **Manage stress:** Practice relaxation techniques like yoga, meditation, or deep breathing to lower stress levels.

- **Regular exercise:** Physical activity helps reduce inflammation and enhances overall health.

- **Maintain a healthy weight:** Excess weight can increase inflammation, so

Copyrighted Material

prioritize weight management through diet and exercise.

- **Adequate sleep:** Sleep deprivation can contribute to inflammation, so aim for 7-8 hours of sleep each night.

- **Seek medical advice:** If concerned about chronic inflammation, consult your doctor to rule out underlying medical conditions.

Remember: Chronic inflammation is a serious health threat, but it's not inevitable. By proactively reducing inflammation, we can safeguard our health. Fuel your body with nourishing foods, stay active, manage stress, and prioritize sleep. Together, we can extinguish the flames of chronic inflammation and build a foundation for vibrant health.

Copyrighted Material

How Anti-Inflammatory Diets Can Be a Game-Changer

In the realm of well-being, the rise of anti-inflammatory diets stands as a transformative game-changer. These dietary strategies hold the promise of transforming health outcomes and safeguarding individuals from the harmful impacts of chronic inflammation. Let's delve into how anti-inflammatory diets can redefine the game:

- **Tackling Chronic Inflammation:** Crafted to extinguish the fires of chronic inflammation, anti-inflammatory diets target the root cause of various health issues. By purposefully choosing foods that combat inflammation, individuals can liberate themselves from the ongoing activation of the immune system.

Copyrighted Material

- **Fortification Against Diseases:** A game-changer in disease prevention, anti-inflammatory diets have been linked to a reduced risk of conditions such as heart disease, cancer, and autoimmune disorders. Addressing inflammation at its core, these diets serve as a powerful defense against a spectrum of illnesses.

- **Balancing the Body's Response:** Striving for equilibrium in the body's inflammatory response, these diets incorporate nutrient-rich foods, omega-3 fatty acids, and antioxidants. This balance promotes overall health and well-being, fostering a state of internal harmony.

- **Boosting Mental Health:** Beyond physical benefits, anti-inflammatory diets extend their positive impact on mental health. Research indicates a correlation

Copyrighted Material

between inflammation and conditions such as depression and anxiety. By embracing an anti-inflammatory approach, individuals may witness favorable effects on mood and cognitive function.

- **Enhancing Overall Well-Being:** Anti-inflammatory diets transcend mere dietary preferences, embodying a holistic approach to well-being. Encouraging the consumption of whole, unprocessed foods and advocating for a balanced lifestyle, these diets lay the groundwork for sustained health and vitality.

Ready to Play the Game?

- **Start Small:** Begin by incorporating small changes into your diet. Add a colorful salad to your lunch or swap sugary snacks for nuts and seeds. The key is gradual progress.

Copyrighted Material

- **Focus on Variety:** Fill your plate with a diverse range of fruits, vegetables, and whole grains, and experiment with healthy fats and spices. Variety provides a diverse range of nutrients.

- **Make it Delicious:** Anti-inflammatory food doesn't have to be bland. Explore new recipes, discover flavorful herbs and spices, and cook with fresh, seasonal ingredients to make your meals a delightful experience.

- **Listen to Your Body:** Be mindful of how your body responds to specific foods. If you notice signs of inflammation or discomfort, adapt your choices accordingly. The journey is about discovering what suits you best and aligning your dietary preferences with your individual well-being.

Copyrighted Material

The Game-Changing Impact:

Adopting an anti-inflammatory diet and lifestyle will result in a significant improvement in your health:

- **Increased Energy:** Inflammation affects your vitality; lowering it makes you feel more energized and ready to face the day.

- **Better Mood:** Chronic inflammation has been related to sadness and anxiety. Fighting inflammation may improve your mood and emotional well-being.

- **Reduced pain and discomfort:** Aches and pains are common manifestations of inflammation. Controlling inflammation allows you to find respite and go through life more comfortably.

- **Improved Immunity:** A balanced anti-inflammatory diet boosts your

Copyrighted Material

immune system, making you more resistant to infections and sickness.

- **Weight management:** Inflammation may cause weight gain. Reducing inflammation may make it simpler for you to maintain a healthy weight.

The Takeaway:

Anti-inflammatory food is more than just a fad; it is a game changer for your health and happiness. It's about making educated decisions, fueling your body with tasty and powerful foods, and enabling yourself to live a life free of chronic inflammation. So take your shopping bag, lace up your shoes, and start your anti-inflammatory journey. Remember that you are the chef, fighter, and ruler of your own health.

Copyrighted Material

CHAPTER 2: BUILDING YOUR CULINARY ARSENAL

Selecting Premium Ingredients for Optimal Nutrition

Embarking on your anti-inflammatory journey extends beyond mere recipes and techniques; it commences with a crucial foundation – your ingredients. Think of them as your weaponry in the war against inflammation, each selection made meticulously for both potency and flavor. Let's delve into the realm of premium ingredients and arm yourself with the finest!

Embracing Freshness:

- **Fruits and Vegetables:** Give precedence to organic produce when available. Locally sourced, in-season fruits and

Copyrighted Material

vegetables boast peak concentrations of vitamins, minerals, and anti-inflammatory compounds. Look for vibrant colors, and firm textures, and explore heirloom varieties for unique flavor profiles.

- **Herbs and Spices:** Fresh herbs like rosemary, thyme, and cilantro add a burst of flavor and a dose of antioxidants. Invest in a small herb garden or visit your local farmers' market for the freshest options. Opt for whole spices and grind them for maximum aroma and flavor.

Protein Excellence:

- **Fish and Seafood:** Opt for wild-caught salmon, sardines, and mackerel, rich in omega-3 fatty acids, and potent anti-inflammatory agents. Consider sustainably sourced options for ethical considerations.

Copyrighted Material

- **Eggs:** Choose pasture-raised eggs for elevated levels of omega-3s and vitamin D, both beneficial for inflammation reduction.

- **Legumes:** Opt for organic, dried varieties of lentils, beans, and chickpeas, rich in plant-based protein and fiber, contributing to gut health and inflammation control.

Healthy Fats:

- **Olive Oil:** Make extra virgin olive oil, cold-pressed and unrefined, a cornerstone for anti-inflammatory cooking. Its monounsaturated fats and antioxidants make it a heart-healthy choice.

- **Nuts and Seeds:** Almonds, walnuts, chia seeds, and flaxseeds are packed with healthy fats, fiber, and anti-inflammatory compounds. Sprinkle them on salads, or

Copyrighted Material

yogurt, or incorporate them into baked goods.

- **Avocado:** This creamy fruit offers a delectable source of healthy fats, fiber, and potassium, contributing to overall well-being and inflammation reduction.

Superfood Squad:

- **Berries:** Blueberries, raspberries, and strawberries emerge as antioxidant powerhouses, aiding in inflammation combat and cell protection. Freeze them for smoothies or relish them fresh as a healthy snack.

- **Turmeric:** With curcumin as its star, this vibrant spice boasts potent anti-inflammatory properties. Integrate it into curries, stir-fries, or even homemade turmeric lattes.

Copyrighted Material

- **Garlic and Ginger:** These flavorful ingredients not only add depth but also possess anti-inflammatory properties. Utilize them fresh or in powdered form for optimal benefits.

Beyond the Essentials:

- **Fermented Foods:** Kombucha, kimchi, and yogurt with live cultures are rich in probiotics, beneficial bacteria that support gut health and potentially reducing inflammation.

- **Organic Broths and Stocks:** Homemade or premium organic broths and stocks form a flavorful foundation for soups and stews, adding nutrients and elevating the anti-inflammatory potential of your meals.

- **Herbal Teas:** Green tea, chamomile, and ginger tea provide a soothing and

Copyrighted Material

delightful way to hydrate while reaping the benefits of anti-inflammatory herbs.

Remember: Premium ingredients are not just about price; it's about quality, freshness, and supporting sustainable practices. Invest in the best you can afford, and relish not only in delightful flavors but also in the assurance that you're arming your body with potent anti-inflammatory weapons.

So, armed with this knowledge, explore local markets, and construct a culinary arsenal that's both delectable and health-promoting. Your anti-inflammatory journey awaits, and with these superior ingredients, you're well on your path to a vibrant, healthy life!

Copyrighted Material

Unveiling the Must-Have Tools and Gadgets in Your Kitchen

Your anti-inflammatory culinary journey extends beyond ingredients. To truly master the kitchen and keep inflammation at bay, it requires the right tools and gadgets as your loyal allies. Think of them as essential companions, aiding you in transforming fresh produce into delightful and health-promoting meals. Let's explore the indispensable weapons in your anti-inflammatory arsenal:

Chopping Champions:

- **Sharp Knives:** Non-negotiable essentials include a quality chef's knife and a smaller paring knife. Invest in sharp knives for effortless chopping of fruits, vegetables, and herbs.

Copyrighted Material

- **Mandoline Slicer:** A game-changer for uniform slices and julienne cuts. Opt for one with adjustable thickness and safety features.

- **Spiralizer:** Transform vegetables into healthy noodles with ease. A spiralizer adds a fun twist to your culinary creations.

Cooking Essentials:

- **High-Quality Skillet:** Choose a cast-iron or stainless steel skillet for searing, sautéing, and stir-frying. Opt for one with good heat distribution for consistent cooking.

- **Dutch Oven:** Versatile for simmering soups, stews, and sauces. Look for one with a tight-fitting lid to retain moisture and flavor.

- **Steamer Basket:** Preserve nutrients by steaming vegetables. A collapsible

Copyrighted Material

steamer basket fits most pots and is easy to store.

Blending Efficiency:

- **High-Powered Blender:** Blend smoothies, purees, and sauces effortlessly. Seek one with multiple settings and durable blades.

- **Food Processor:** Ideal for chopping nuts, shredding vegetables, and making various dishes. Consider a model with interchangeable blades for versatility.

Hydration Essentials:

- **Reusable Water Bottle:** Stay hydrated with a stylish and practical reusable water bottle. Opt for stainless steel or glass for a healthier and eco-friendly choice.

- **Infuser Pitcher:** Add a refreshing twist to your water with fruits, herbs, or cucumber.

Copyrighted Material

An infuser pitcher simplifies the process and keeps floating bits at bay.

Bonus Kitchen Gadgets:

- **Spiralizer for Nuts and Seeds:** Elevate your dishes with homemade nut butter and seed flour. A dedicated nut and seed spiralizer ensures safety and efficiency.

- **Herb Keeper:** Extend the life of fresh herbs like basil and cilantro with a herb keeper, providing water and preventing wilting.

- **Microplane Grater:** This fine grater unlocks intense flavors of citrus zest, ginger, and garlic. Add a touch of culinary magic to your dishes.

Remember: Choose tools that align with your cooking style and needs. Focus on quality and versatility rather than overwhelming yourself with an abundance of appliances. As you embark

Copyrighted Material

on your anti-inflammatory journey, discover which tools become your trusted companions in the kitchen.

So, equip yourself with this arsenal of culinary helpers, unleash your inner chef, and relish the process of crafting delicious and health-promoting meals. Remember, the right tools can make all the difference in your anti-inflammatory kitchen adventures!

Smart Shopping Strategies for Anti-Inflammatory Eating

Embarking on your anti-inflammatory journey isn't just about fancy gadgets and trendy superfoods; it's about wise grocery choices, navigating the path like a seasoned warrior against inflammation. Grab your reusable bag,

Copyrighted Material

and let's uncover strategies for a triumphant and budget-friendly anti-inflammatory shopping spree:

Plan Ahead:

- **Weekly Meal Plan:** Sketch out your weekly meals to avoid impulsive purchases and guarantee you possess the right ingredients for anti-inflammatory culinary creations.

- **Make a List:** Stick to your list, sidestepping distractions. This ensures a focus on anti-inflammatory essentials, preventing unnecessary expenditures.

Prioritize Produce:

- **Seasonal & Local:** Opt for fresh, seasonal fruits and veggies for heightened flavor and nutrients. Supporting local farmers not only benefits your health but also nurtures the community.

Copyrighted Material

- **Variety is Key:** Don't stick to the same old suspects. Explore different colors and textures to ensure you're getting a diverse range of anti-inflammatory vitamins and minerals.

- **Frozen & Canned Allies:** Budget-friendly options in frozen and canned produce provide nutritional perks without unwarranted additives. Select those that don't have any preservatives or extra sugar.

Protein Excellence:

- **Lean & Sustainable:** Lean proteins like chicken, fish, tofu, or lentils are preferred. Choose ethically sourced options whenever available.

- **Plant-Powered Magic:** Beans and lentils, filled up with protein, fiber, and anti-inflammatory compounds, elevate

Copyrighted Material

your culinary repertoire. Diversify with various varieties for versatile meals.

- **Egg Elevation:** Opt for pasture-raised eggs, rich in omega-3s and vitamin D, contributing to inflammation reduction.

Healthy Fats & Culinary Marvels:

- **Olive Oil:** Extra virgin olive oil stands as a cornerstone for anti-inflammatory cooking. Seek cold-pressed, unrefined options for optimal flavor and health benefits.

- **Nuts & Seeds:** Almonds, walnuts, chia seeds, and flaxseeds become treasures for healthy fats, fiber, and anti-inflammatory goodness.

- Superfood Companions: Maintain a small cache of berries, turmeric, ginger, and garlic; these anti-inflammatory heroes not

Copyrighted Material

only enhance flavor but also boost the health of your meals.

Budget-Conscious Choices:

- **Buy in Bulk:** If storage allows, buying staples like beans, grains, and nuts in bulk can yield long-term savings.

- **Store Brand Wisdom:** Store brands often provide comparable nutrition at a more budget-friendly price.

- **Compare Prices:** Assess unit prices and explore weekly flyers for optimal deals. Don't hesitate to switch brands for better value.

Don't Forget the Essentials:

- **Herbs & Spices Symphony:** Fresh herbs and whole spices not only elevate flavor but also enrich your meals with anti-inflammatory benefits. Consider

Copyrighted Material

cultivating your herb garden for a cost-effective option.

- **Broths & Stocks:** Quality broths elevate the flavors of soups and stews while contributing to your anti-inflammatory goals.

- **Herbal Tea Bliss:** Green tea, chamomile, and ginger tea hydrate and delightfully deliver anti-inflammatory benefits.

Bonus Culinary Hacks:

- **Shop at Farmers' Markets:** Connect with local farmers for fresh, seasonal produce at competitive prices.

- **Label Mastery:** Scrutinize ingredients and serving sizes, steering clear of processed foods laden with added sugars, unhealthy fats, and artificial additives.

- **Cook at Home:** By preparing meals at home, you gain control over ingredients

Copyrighted Material

and portions, facilitating adherence to your anti-inflammatory goals.

Remember, smart shopping is an ongoing journey, not a one-time sprint. Experiment, compare, and discover what aligns best with your preferences and budget. Armed with these cookbook-style strategies, conquer the grocery aisles, and fuel your anti-inflammatory journey with delectable and healthful choices!

An Anti-Inflammatory Lifestyle Includes:

- Limiting foods that increase inflammation
- Eating anti-inflammatory foods
- Not smoking
- Limiting alcohol intake
- Being physically active
- Getting enough quality sleep
- Managing Stress
- Managing Weight

Copyrighted Material

CHAPTER 3: BREAKFAST DELIGHTS

Energizing Smoothie Bowls

Tropical Paradise Smoothie Bowl

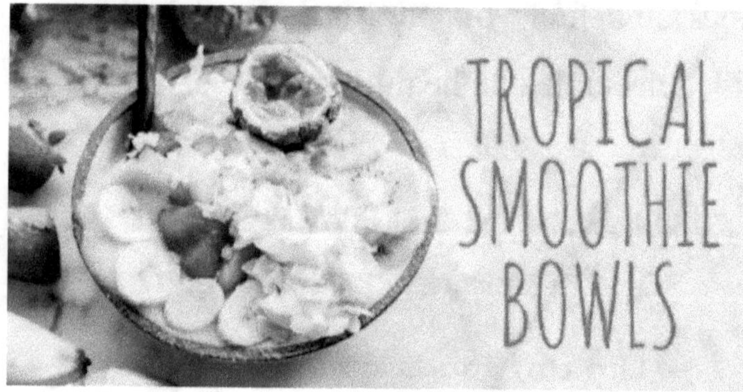

Ingredients:

- 1 cup frozen mango chunks
- 1/2 cup pineapple chunks
- 1/2 banana
- 1/2 cup coconut milk

Copyrighted Material

- 1 tablespoon chia seeds

- 1 tablespoon shredded coconut

Toppings:

- Sliced kiwi

- Granola

- Passion fruit seeds

- Pineapple chunks

- Mint leaves

Preparation:

- Blend mango, pineapple, banana, coconut milk, and chia seeds until smooth.

- Adjust consistency with more coconut milk if needed.

- Pour into a bowl and top with kiwi, granola, passion fruit seeds, pineapple, and mint.

- Dive into the Tropical Paradise Smoothie Bowl and savor the tropical bliss!

Copyrighted Material

Nutritional Value:

- Calories: 380 kcal
- Protein: 5g
- Fat: 15g
- Carbohydrates: 60g
- Fiber: 10g
- Sugar: 35g

Acai Berry Burst Bowl

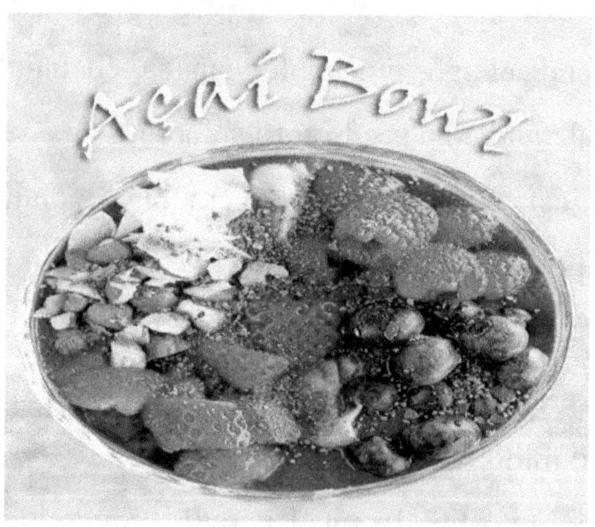

Ingredients:

- 1 packet of frozen acai puree

Copyrighted Material

- 1/2 cup mixed berries
- 1/2 banana
- 1/2 cup almond milk
- 1 tablespoon hemp seeds
- 1 tablespoon almond butter

Toppings:

- Granola
- Sliced strawberries
- Chia seeds
- Sliced almonds
- Drizzle of honey

Preparation:

- Blend acai puree, mixed berries, banana, almond milk, hemp seeds, and almond butter until smooth.
- Adjust consistency with more almond milk if needed.

Copyrighted Material

- Pour into a bowl and top with granola, strawberries, chia seeds, almonds, and a drizzle of honey.
- Indulge in the Acai Berry Burst Bowl for a nutrient-packed breakfast.

Nutritional Value:

- Calories: 420 kcal
- Protein: 10g
- Fat: 20g
- Carbohydrates: 55g
- Fiber: 12g
- Sugar: 30g

Peanut Butter Power Bowl

Copyrighted Material

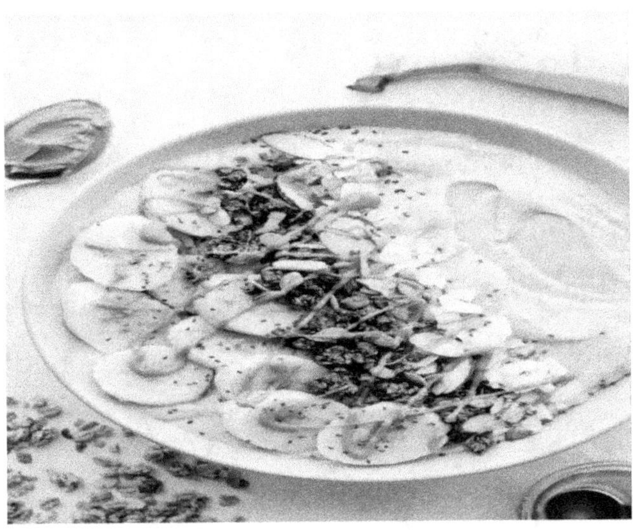

Ingredients:

- 2 frozen bananas

- 2 tablespoons peanut butter

- 1 cup spinach leaves

- 1/2 cup milk

- 1 tablespoon cocoa powder

- 1 tablespoon flaxseeds

Toppings:

- Sliced banana

- Dark chocolate shavings

- Crushed peanuts
- Coconut flakes
- Sprinkle of sea salt

Preparation:

- Blend bananas, peanut butter, spinach, milk, cocoa powder, and flaxseeds until creamy.
- Adjust consistency with more milk if needed.
- Pour into a bowl and top with sliced banana, chocolate shavings, peanuts, coconut flakes, and a sprinkle of sea salt.
- Revel in the Peanut Butter Power Bowl, a protein-rich way to start your day.

Nutritional Value:

- Calories: 400 kcal
- Protein: 12g
- Fat: 15g
- Carbohydrates: 60g

Copyrighted Material

- Fiber: 10g
- Sugar: 30g

These vibrant smoothie bowls offer a spectrum of flavors and nutrients, ensuring a delicious and energizing start to your mornings. Customize ingredients and toppings to suit your taste and dietary preferences.

Anti-Inflammatory Breakfast Wraps

Mediterranean Veggie Wrap

Copyrighted Material

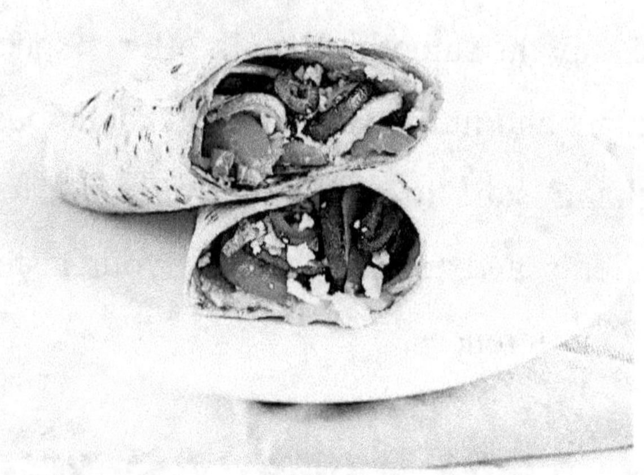

Ingredients:

- Whole-grain or spinach tortilla
- 2 tablespoons hummus
- Sliced cucumber
- Cherry tomatoes
- Kalamata olives
- Red onion
- Feta cheese
- Fresh basil leaves
- Drizzle of olive oil

Copyrighted Material

- Salt and pepper

Preparation:

- Spread hummus on the tortilla.

- Layer cucumber, cherry tomatoes, olives, red onion, feta, and basil.

- Season with salt and pepper after drizzling with olive oil.

- Wrap the tortilla tightly, cut in half, and enjoy this Mediterranean-inspired anti-inflammatory breakfast.

Nutritional Value:

- Calories: 350 kcal

- Protein: 10g

- Fat: 18g

- Carbohydrates: 40g

- Fiber: 8g

- Sugar: 5g

Smoked Salmon Avocado Wrap

Copyrighted Material

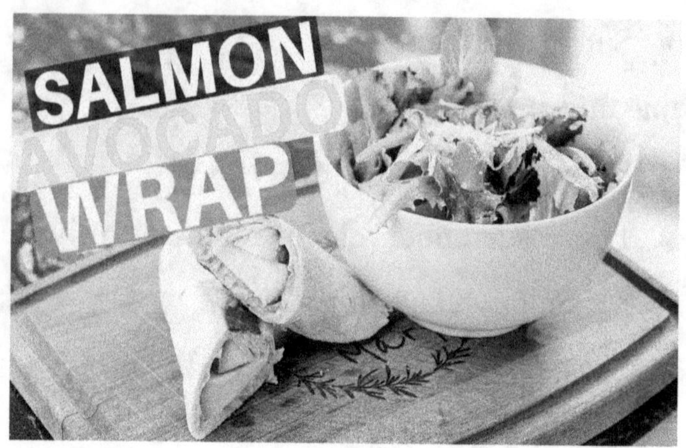

Ingredients:

- Whole-grain or flaxseed tortilla
- 2 tablespoons cream cheese
- Smoked salmon
- Sliced avocado
- Baby spinach
- Capers
- Fresh dill
- Lemon zest
- Salt and pepper

Preparation:

Copyrighted Material

- Spread cream cheese on the tortilla.

- Arrange salmon, avocado, spinach, capers, and dill.

- Add lemon zest and season with salt and pepper.

- Roll, slice, and savor the delightful flavors of this smoked salmon avocado wrap.

Nutritional Value:

- Calories: 380 kcal

- Protein: 20g

- Fat: 22g

- Carbohydrates: 30g

- Fiber: 8g

- Sugar: 2g

Southwestern Black Bean Wrap

Copyrighted Material

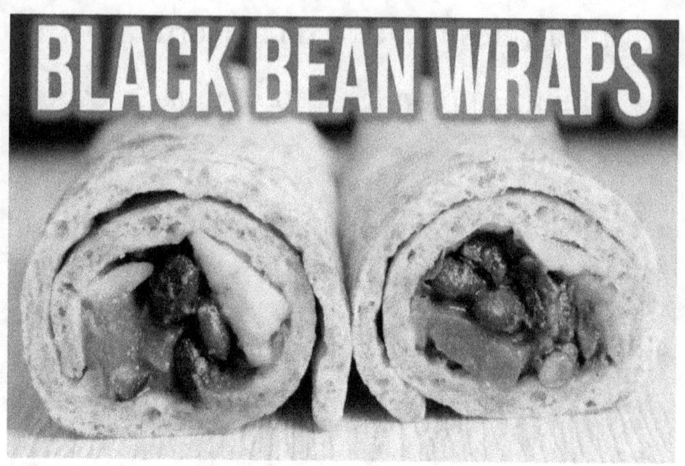

Ingredients:

- Whole-grain or corn tortilla
- 1/2 cup cooked and mashed black beans
- Sliced grilled chicken (optional)
- Salsa
- Bell peppers
- Red onion
- Fresh cilantro
- Lime wedge
- Salt and cumin

Preparation:

Copyrighted Material

- Spread mashed black beans on the tortilla.

- If using, add sliced grilled chicken and mix with salsa.

- Arrange the chopped red onion, sliced bell peppers, and fresh cilantro in layers.

- Add salt and cumin to the ingredients and squeeze a lime wedge over them.

- Enjoy the flavors of this Southwestern black bean wrap by rolling the tortilla, cutting it into half, and eating it.

Nutritional Value:
- Calories: 320 kcal

- Protein: 18g

- Fat: 8g

- Carbohydrates: 45g

- Fiber: 12g

- Sugar: 4g

These anti-inflammatory breakfast wraps not only burst with flavors but also provide a

Copyrighted Material

nutritional boost to kickstart your day. Tailor the ingredients to match your personal preferences and dietary requirements.

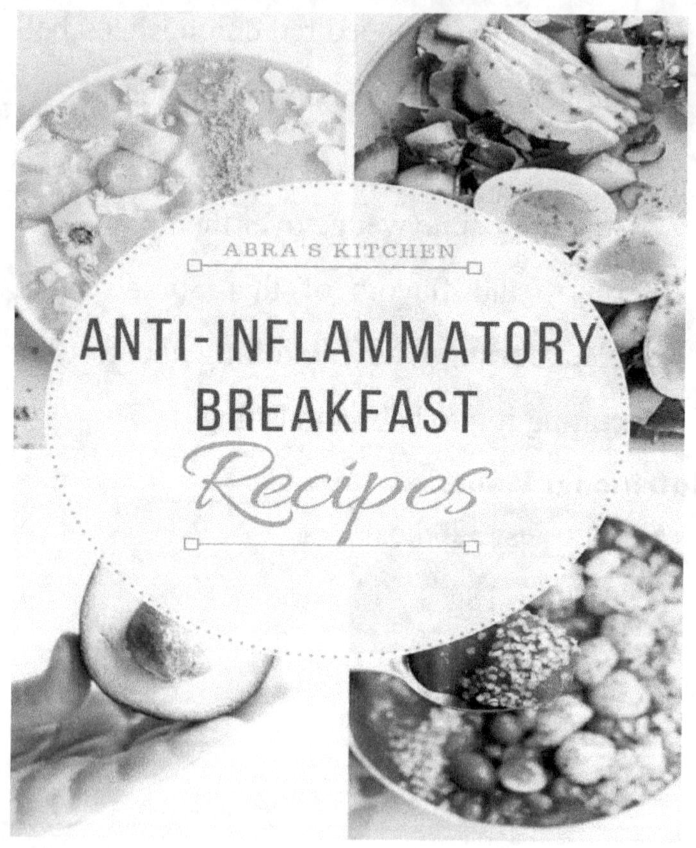

Copyrighted Material

CHAPTER 4: LUNCHTIME FAVORITES

Vibrant Salad Creations

Garden Harvest Salad

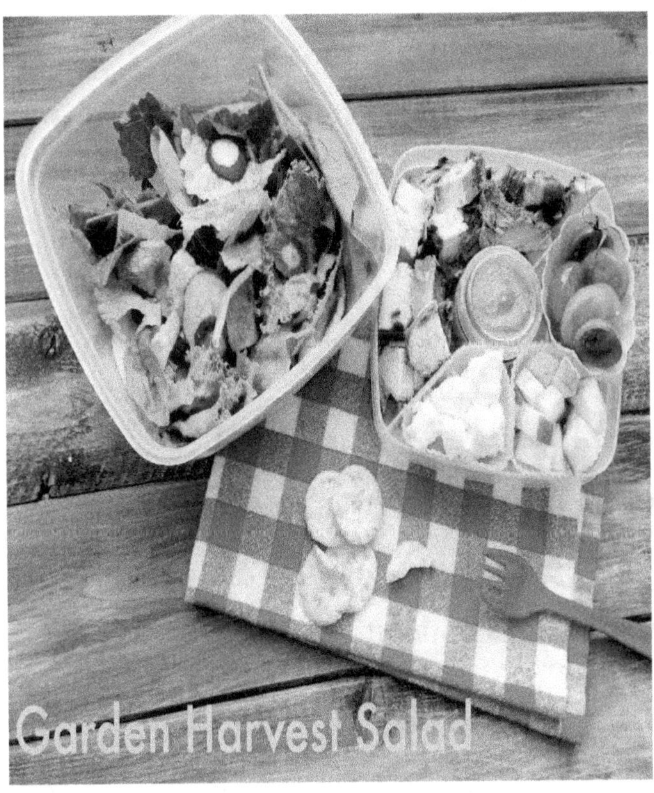

Copyrighted Material

Ingredients:

Salad:

- 4 cups mixed salad greens

- 1 cup cherry tomatoes, halved

- 1 cucumber, sliced

- 1/2 red onion, thinly sliced

- 1 cup shredded carrots

- 1/2 cup radishes, thinly sliced

- 1/4 cup crumbled goat cheese

- 1/4 cup sunflower seeds

Balsamic Vinaigrette:

- 3 tablespoons balsamic vinegar

- 1/4 cup extra-virgin olive oil

- 1 teaspoon Dijon mustard

- 1 clove garlic, minced

- Salt and pepper to taste

Copyrighted Material

Preparation:

- Combine salad greens, cherry tomatoes, cucumber, red onion, shredded carrots, radishes, goat cheese, and sunflower seeds in a large bowl.

- Whisk together balsamic vinegar, olive oil, Dijon mustard, minced garlic, salt, and pepper to create the vinaigrette.

- After drizzling the salad with the vinaigrette, gently toss to coat.

- Serve immediately to enjoy a vivid and fresh Garden Harvest Salad.

Nutritional Value:

- Calories: 320 kcal
- Protein: 8g
- Fat: 25g
- Carbohydrates: 20g
- Fiber: 5g
- Sugar: 8g

Copyrighted Material

Citrus Avocado Quinoa Salad

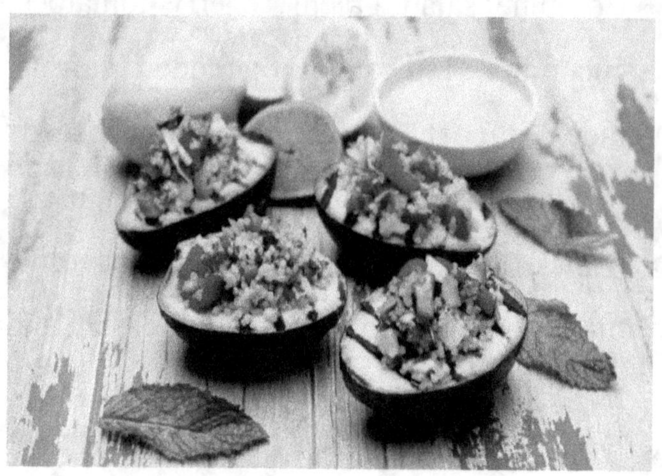

Ingredients:

Salad:

- 2 cups cooked quinoa
- 1 orange, peeled and segmented
- 1 grapefruit, peeled and segmented
- 1 avocado, diced
- 1/4 cup red onion, finely chopped
- 1/4 cup fresh cilantro, chopped
- 1/4 cup pistachios, chopped
- Mixed salad greens for serving

Copyrighted Material

Citrus Dressing:

- Juice of 1 lemon
- Juice of 1 lime
- 2 tablespoons olive oil
- 1 teaspoon honey
- Salt and pepper to taste

Preparation:

- Combine cooked quinoa, orange segments, grapefruit segments, diced avocado, red onion, cilantro, and pistachios in a large bowl.

- Whisk together lemon juice, lime juice, olive oil, honey, salt, and pepper to create the citrus dressing in a small bowl.

- After adding the dressing, gently toss the quinoa mixture.

- Serve the Citrus Avocado Quinoa Salad over a bed of mixed salad greens for a colorful and zesty meal.

Copyrighted Material

Nutritional Value:

- Calories: 380 kcal
- Protein: 10g
- Fat: 18g
- Carbohydrates: 50g
- Fiber: 10g
- Sugar: 8g

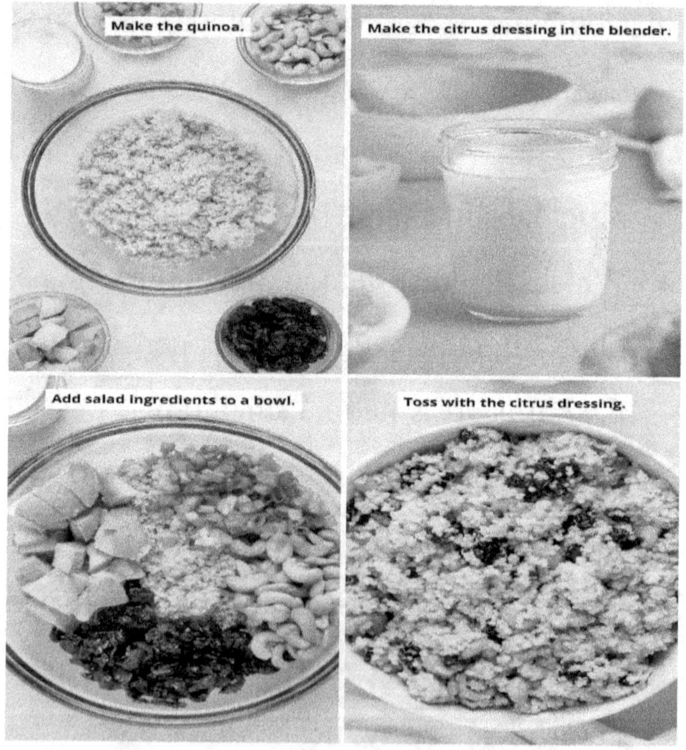

Copyrighted Material

Grilled Peach and Burrata Salad

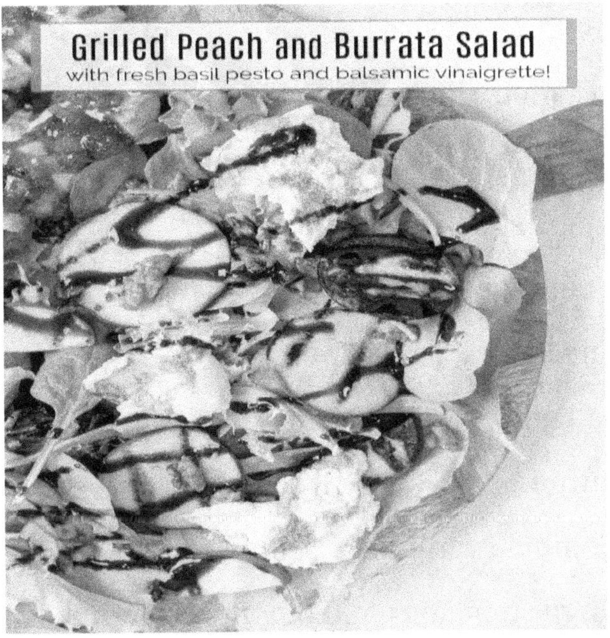

Ingredients:

Salad:

- 4 cups arugula
- 2 ripe peaches, sliced and grilled
- 1/2 cup cherry tomatoes, halved

Copyrighted Material

- 1/4 cup red onion, thinly sliced
- 1/4 cup fresh basil leaves
- 1/4 cup balsamic glaze
- 1 burrata cheese ball, torn into pieces

Honey-Lemon Vinaigrette:

- 3 tablespoons extra-virgin olive oil
- 1 tablespoon balsamic vinegar
- 1 tablespoon honey
- Juice of 1 lemon
- Salt and pepper to taste

Preparation:

- Combine arugula, grilled peach slices, cherry tomatoes, red onion, and fresh basil leaves in a large bowl.
- Drizzle balsamic glaze over the salad and toss gently.

Copyrighted Material

- Whisk together olive oil, balsamic vinegar, honey, lemon juice, salt, and pepper to create the vinaigrette.

- After adding the vinaigrette, mix the salad to coat.

- Top the salad with torn burrata pieces and serve the Grilled Peach and Burrata Salad as a delightful and sophisticated dish.

Nutritional Value:

- Calories: 320 kcal

- Protein: 8g

- Fat: 25g

- Carbohydrates: 20g

- Fiber: 5g

- Sugar: 12g

These vibrant salads offer a delightful combination of flavors, textures, and nutrients.

Copyrighted Material

Customize the recipes to suit your taste and enjoy these colorful and nutritious meals.

Flavorful Grain Bowls

Mediterranean Quinoa Bowl

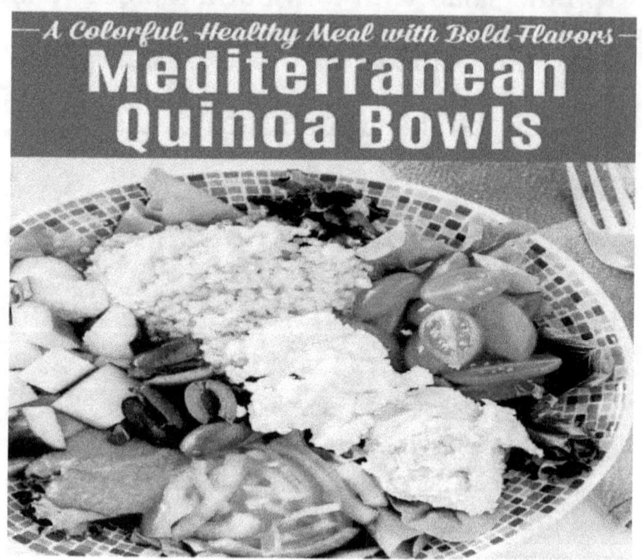

Ingredients:

Grain Bowl:

- 1 cup cooked quinoa
- 1/2 cup chickpeas, cooked and seasoned

Copyrighted Material

- 1/2 cup cherry tomatoes, halved
- 1/4 cup cucumber, diced
- 1/4 cup Kalamata olives, sliced
- 1/4 cup red onion, finely chopped
- Feta cheese, crumbled
- Fresh parsley for garnish

Lemon-Herb Dressing:

- 3 tablespoons extra-virgin olive oil
- Juice of 1 lemon
- 1 teaspoon dried oregano
- Salt and pepper to taste

Preparation:

- Place the cooked quinoa, chopped red onion, diced cucumber, sliced Kalamata olives, feta cheese, cherry tomatoes, and seasoned chickpeas in a bowl.
- To make the dressing, combine the olive oil, lemon juice, dried oregano, salt, and pepper in a small container.

Copyrighted Material

- Add some fresh parsley as a garnish and drizzle the dressing over the grain dish.
- Gently toss and enjoy this Quinoa Bowl's Mediterranean flavors.

Nutritional Value:

- Calories: 380 kcal
- Protein: 12g
- Fat: 18g
- Carbohydrates: 45g
- Fiber: 8g
- Sugar: 4g

Teriyaki Salmon and Brown Rice Bowl

Copyrighted Material

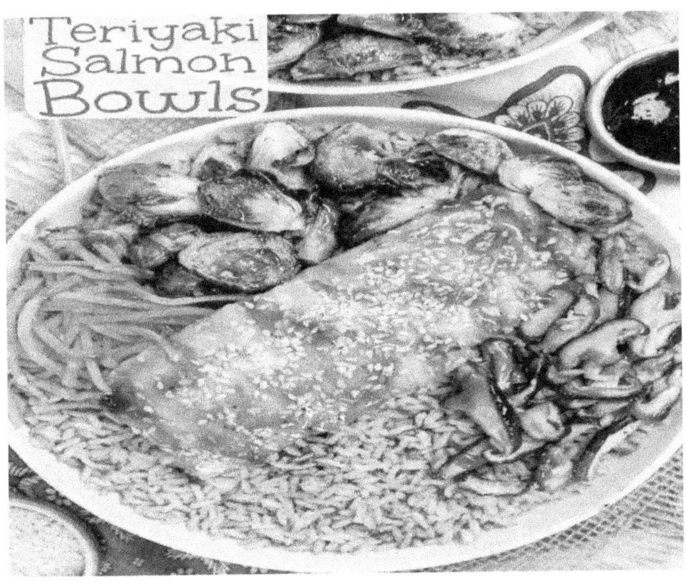

Ingredients:

Grain Bowl:

- 1 cup cooked brown rice
- 6 ounces salmon filet, grilled or baked with teriyaki glaze
- 1/2 cup broccoli florets, steamed
- 1/2 cup carrot, julienned and sautéed
- 1/4 cup edamame, steamed

Copyrighted Material

- Sesame seeds for garnish
- Sliced green onions for garnish

Teriyaki Glaze:

- 2 tablespoons soy sauce
- 1 tablespoon honey
- 1 teaspoon rice vinegar
- 1/2 teaspoon sesame oil
- 1/2 teaspoon grated ginger
- 1 clove garlic, minced

Preparation:

- Put cooked brown rice in a bowl and top with grilled or baked teriyaki salmon.
- Mix in steamed broccoli, sautéed julienned carrots, and steamed edamame.
- To make the teriyaki glaze, whisk together soy sauce, honey, rice vinegar, sesame oil, grated ginger, and chopped garlic.

Copyrighted Material

- Drizzle the glaze over the veggies and fish.
- Sprinkle it with sesame seeds and sliced green onions.
- For a delicious and filling supper, enjoy the Teriyaki Salmon and Brown Rice Bowl.

Nutritional Value:

- Calories: 450 kcal
- Protein: 25g
- Fat: 15g
- Carbohydrates: 55g
- Fiber: 8g
- Sugar: 10g

Mexican-Inspired Quinoa Bowl

Copyrighted Material

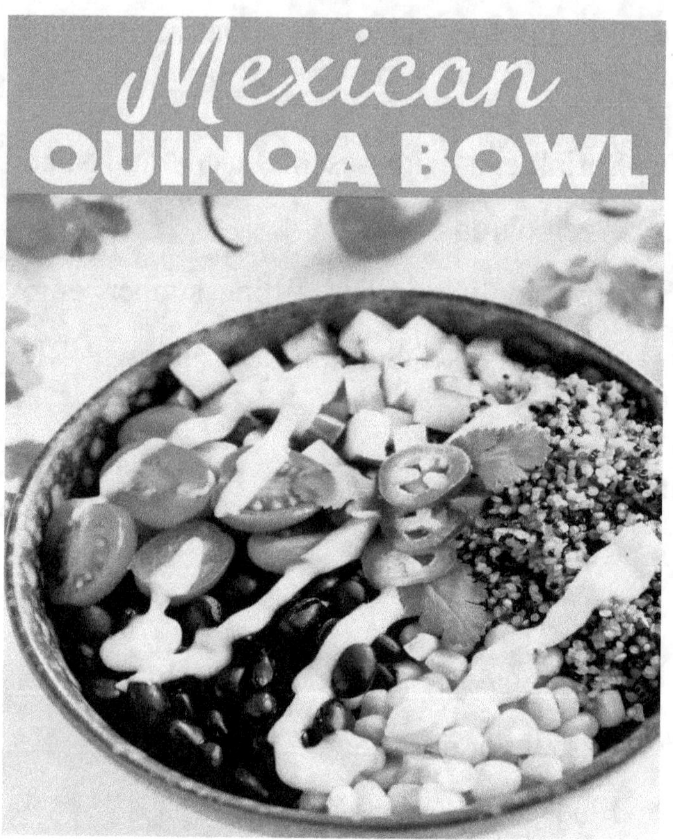

Ingredients:

Grain Bowl:

- 1 cup cooked quinoa

- 1/2 cup black beans, cooked and seasoned

- 1/2 cup corn kernels, grilled or sautéed

Copyrighted Material

- 1/4 cup cherry tomatoes, halved
- 1/4 cup red onion, finely chopped
- Avocado slices
- Fresh cilantro for garnish

Chipotle-Lime Dressing:

- 3 tablespoons Greek yogurt
- Juice of 1 lime
- 1 teaspoon of canned chipotle peppers' adobo sauce
- 1/2 teaspoon ground cumin
- Salt and pepper to taste

Preparation:

- In a bowl, combine the cooked quinoa, seasoned black beans, grilled corn kernels, cherry tomatoes, chopped red onion, and avocado slices.

Copyrighted Material

- Combine Greek yogurt, lime juice, adobo sauce, ground cumin, salt, and pepper to make the chipotle-lime dressing.
- Drizzle the dressing over the grain dish, then top with fresh cilantro.
- Toss gently and enjoy the vibrant flavors of this Mexican-inspired Quinoa Bowl.

Nutritional Value:
- Calories: 380 kcal
- Protein: 12g
- Fat: 18g
- Carbohydrates: 45g
- Fiber: 10g
- Sugar: 4g

These flavorful grain bowls provide a satisfying and nourishing experience. Customize the recipes to suit your taste and dietary preferences for a delicious and wholesome meal.

Copyrighted Material

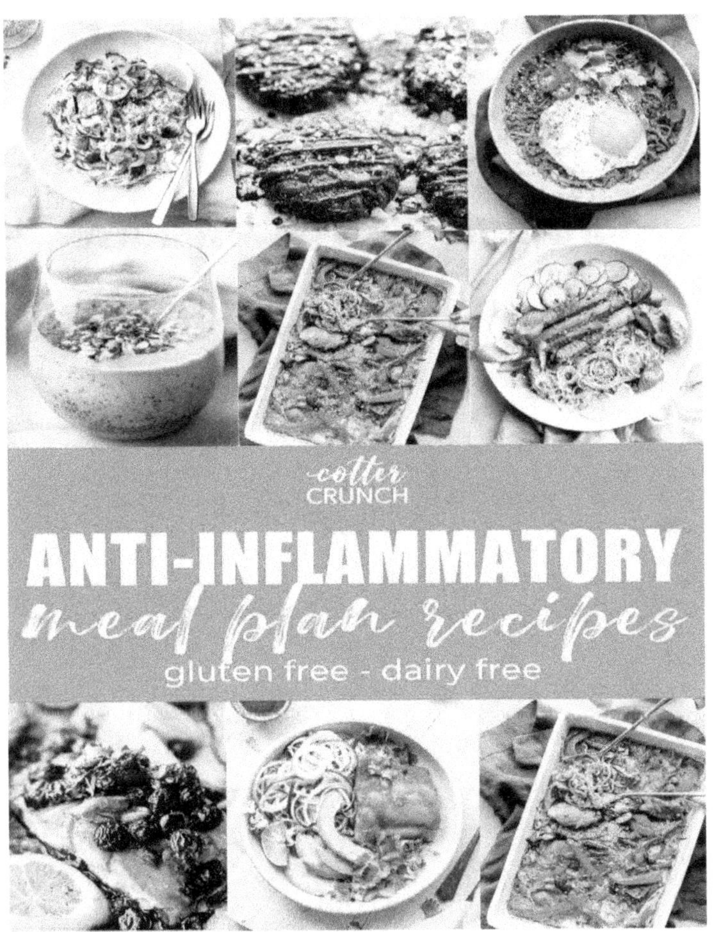

Copyrighted Material

CHAPTER 5: DINNER DELICACIES

Satisfying One-Pot Wonders

Tuscan White Bean and Kale Stew

Copyrighted Material

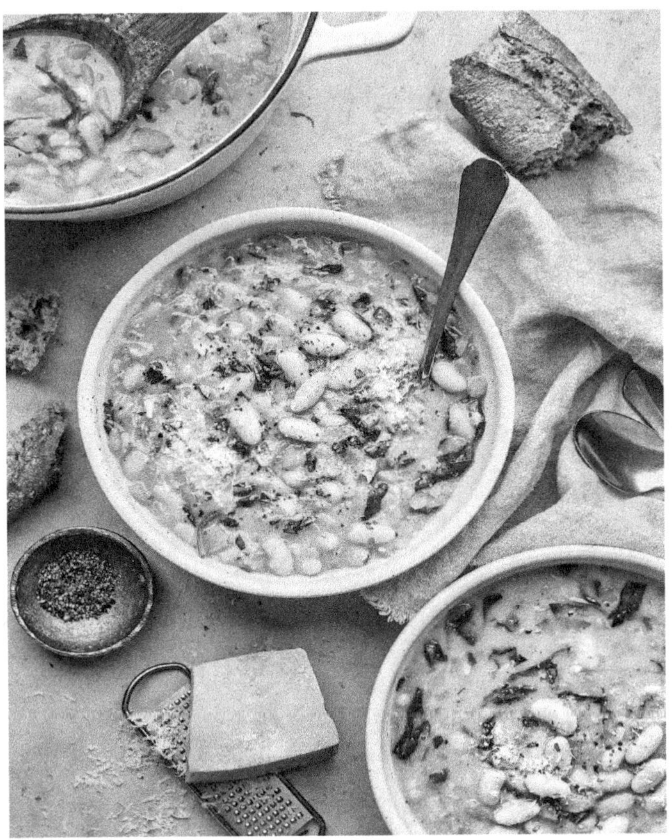

Ingredients:

- 1 tbsp olive oil

- 1 onion, diced

- 3 cloves garlic, minced

- 2 carrots, sliced

Copyrighted Material

- 2 celery stalks, chopped
- 1 can (15 ounces) of drained white beans
- 1 can (14 oz) diced tomatoes
- 4 cups vegetable broth
- 1 tsp dried thyme
- 1 tsp dried rosemary
- 1 bay leaf
- Salt and pepper to taste
- 2 cups kale, chopped
- Grated Parmesan for serving

Preparation:

- In a large pot, warm the olive oil over medium heat. Mix in diced onion, minced garlic, sliced carrots, and chopped celery. Saute until the vegetables soften.

- Mix in the white beans, chopped tomatoes, vegetable broth, dried thyme, dry rosemary, bay leaf, salt, and pepper.

Copyrighted Material

- Simmer the stew and let it cook for 20-25 minutes.

- To the saucepan, add the chopped kale and cook until wilted.

- Before serving, remove the bay leaf.

- Transfer the Tuscan White Bean and Kale Stew into a bowl and top with grated Parmesan.

Nutritional Value:

- Calories: 280 kcal

- Protein: 12g

- Fat: 5g

- Carbs: 50g

- Fiber: 12g

- Sugar: 8g

Spicy Chickpea and Vegetable Curry

Copyrighted Material

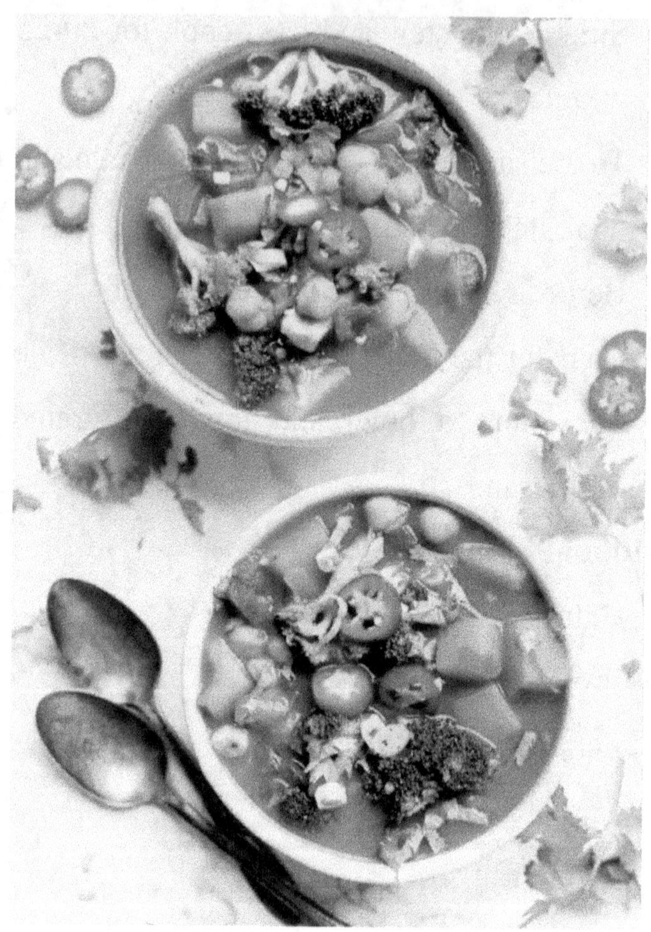

Ingredients:

- 1 tbsp coconut oil

- 1 onion, finely chopped

- 3 cloves garlic, minced

Copyrighted Material

- 1 tbsp ginger, grated
- 2 tbsp curry powder
- 1 tsp ground cumin
- 1 tsp ground coriander
- 1 can (15 oz) chickpeas, drained
- 1 can (14 oz) diced tomatoes
- 1 can (14 oz) coconut milk
- 2 cups mixed vegetables
- Salt and pepper to taste
- Fresh cilantro for garnish
- Cooked basmati rice for serving

Preparation

- Heat coconut oil, sauté onion, garlic, and ginger until onion is translucent.
- Add curry powder, cumin, and coriander. Cook for 1-2 minutes.
- Stir in chickpeas, diced tomatoes, coconut milk, mixed vegetables, salt, and pepper.

Copyrighted Material

- Simmer the curry for 20-25 minutes until vegetables are tender.
- Serve the Spicy Chickpea and Vegetable Curry over cooked basmati rice, garnished with fresh cilantro.

Nutritional Value:

- Calories: 320 kcal
- Protein: 10g
- Fat: 18g
- Carbs: 35g
- Fiber: 8g
- Sugar: 6g

Hearty Lentil and Vegetable Stew

Copyrighted Material

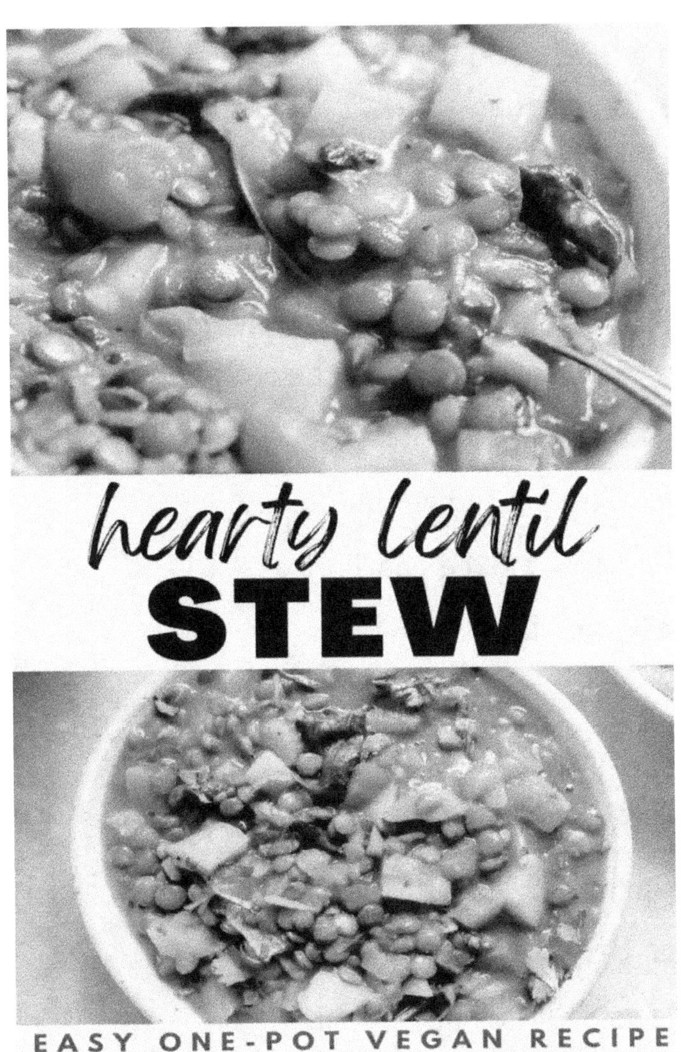

Ingredients:

- 1 tbsp olive oil

Copyrighted Material

- 1 onion, diced

- 2 carrots, sliced

- 2 celery stalks, chopped

- 3 cloves garlic, minced

- 1 cup dry green or brown lentils, rinsed

- 1 can (14 oz) crushed tomatoes

- 6 cups vegetable broth

- 1 tsp ground cumin

- 1 tsp smoked paprika

- 1 bay leaf

- Salt and pepper to taste

- 2 cups baby spinach

- Fresh parsley for garnish

Preparation:

- Heat olive oil, sauté onion, carrots, celery, and garlic until softened.

Copyrighted Material

- Add lentils, crushed tomatoes, vegetable broth, cumin, smoked paprika, bay leaf, salt, and pepper.

- Boil the stew, then reduce heat and simmer for 25-30 minutes until lentils are tender.

- Stir in baby spinach until wilted.

- Remove bay leaf before serving, garnish with parsley.

Nutritional Value:

- Calories: 280 kcal

- Protein: 15g

- Fat: 5g

- Carbs: 45g

- Fiber: 12g

- Sugar: 8g

Copyrighted Material

Oven-Baked Goodness

Baked Lemon Garlic Herb Salmon

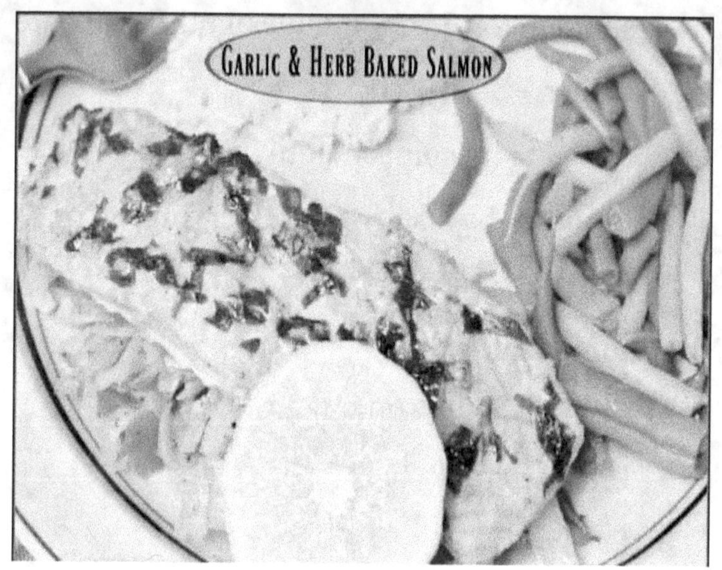

Ingredients:

- 4 salmon filets
- 2 tbsp olive oil
- 3 cloves garlic, minced
- Zest of 1 lemon

Copyrighted Material

- Juice of 1 lemon

- 1 tsp dried thyme

- 1 tsp dried rosemary

- Salt and pepper to taste

- Fresh parsley for garnish

Preparation:

- Preheat the oven to 400°F (200°C).

- Place salmon on a parchment-lined baking sheet.

- Mix olive oil, garlic, lemon zest, lemon juice, thyme, rosemary, salt, and pepper.

- Brush mixture over salmon.

- Bake in the preheated oven for 12-15 minutes or until the salmon is cooked through.

- Garnish with fresh parsley.

Nutritional Value:

- Calories: 300 kcal

Copyrighted Material

- Protein: 30g
- Fat: 18g
- Carbs: 2g
- Fiber: 1g
- Sugar: 0g

Baked Mediterranean Chicken with Vegetables

Copyrighted Material

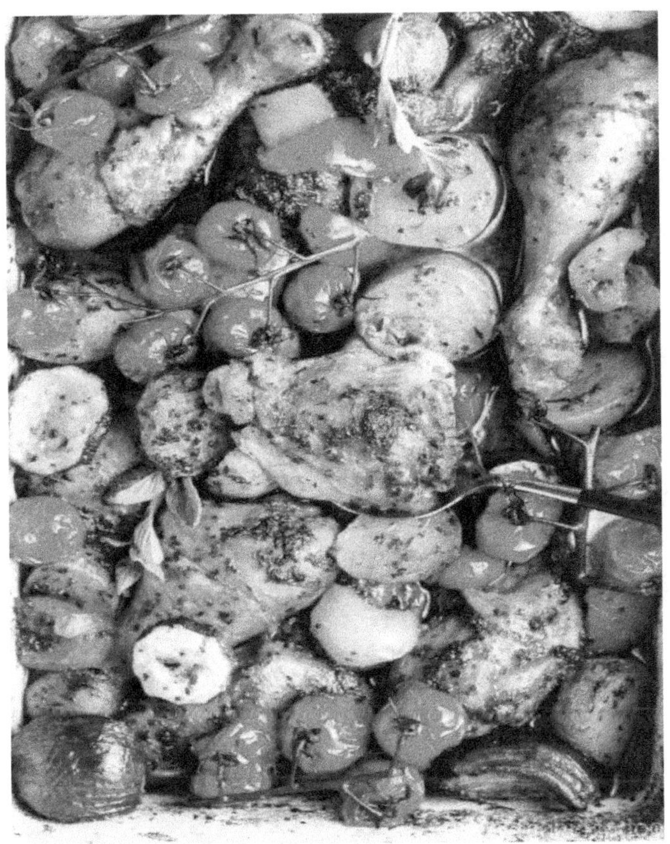

Ingredients:

- 4 boneless, skinless chicken breasts
- 1 cup cherry tomatoes, halved
- 1 cup baby potatoes, halved
- 1/2 cup Kalamata olives, sliced

Copyrighted Material

- 2 tbsp olive oil

- 2 tsp dried oregano

- 1 tsp dried thyme

- 1 tsp garlic powder

- Salt and pepper to taste

- Fresh parsley for garnish

Preparation:

- Set oven temperature to 400°F, or 200°C.

- Arrange baby potatoes, cherry tomatoes, and Kalamata olives on one side of a baking sheet and place chicken breasts on the other side.

- Combine olive oil, garlic powder, salt, pepper, dried oregano, and dried thyme in a small bowl.

- Coat the chicken and veggies with the olive oil mixture.

Copyrighted Material

- Bake for 25 to 30 minutes, or until the chicken is well cooked and the veggies are soft, in a preheated oven.

- Before serving, top the cooked chicken and veggies with crumbled feta cheese and fresh parsley.

Nutritional Value:

- Calories: 380 kcal

- Protein: 30g

- Fat: 16g

- Carbs: 25g

- Fiber: 4g

- Sugar: 3g

Roasted Vegetable and Chickpea Quinoa Bowl

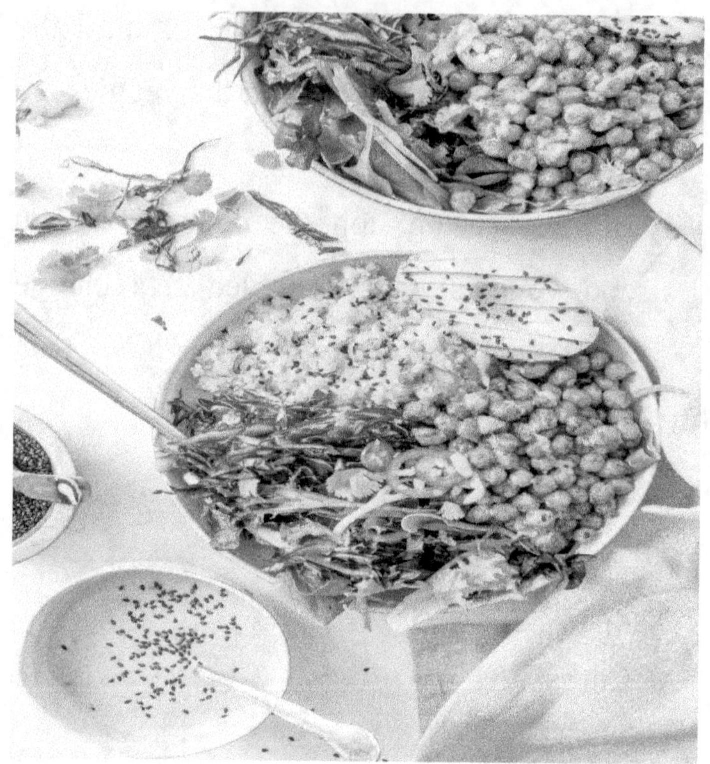

Ingredients:

- 1 cup quinoa, rinsed
- 2 cups broccoli florets
- 1 red bell pepper, sliced
- 1 yellow bell pepper, sliced
- 1 zucchini, sliced
- 1 can (15 oz) chickpeas, drained

Copyrighted Material

- 3 tbsp olive oil

- 1 tsp smoked paprika

- 1 tsp cumin

- 1 tsp garlic powder

- Salt and pepper to taste

- Lemon wedges for serving

Preparation:

- Set the oven temperature to 425°F (220°C).

- Combine the broccoli florets, red bell pepper, yellow bell pepper, garlic powder, cumin, smoked paprika, olive oil, and salt and pepper in a big bowl.

- Transfer the mixture of vegetables and chickpeas onto a baking sheet.

- Roast the veggies for 20 to 25 minutes in a preheated oven, or until they are soft and start to caramelize.

Copyrighted Material

- Prepare the quinoa per the directions on the box while the veggies roast.
- Toss in the quinoa and serve the roasted vegetable and chickpea combination. Garnish with lemon wedges.

Nutritional Value:

- Calories: 420 kcal
- Protein: 15g
- Fat: 16g
- Carbs: 60g
- Fiber: 12g
- Sugar: 4g

Copyrighted Material

CHAPTER 6: SNACKS AND APPETIZERS

Nourishing Nut Mixes

Spiced Maple Pecan Mix

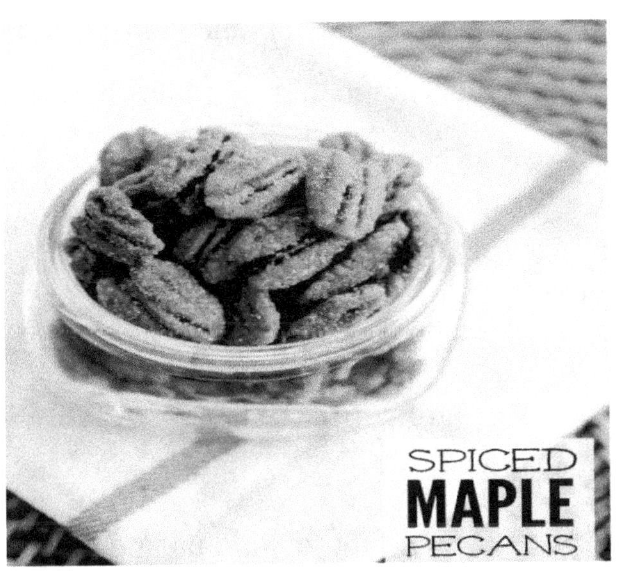

Ingredients:

- 1 cup pecan halves

- 1 cup walnuts

- 1 tablespoon maple syrup

Copyrighted Material

- 1 teaspoon ground cinnamon
- 1/4 teaspoon ground nutmeg
- 1/4 teaspoon sea salt

Preparation:

- Set the oven's temperature to 175°C/350°F.
- Toss pecans and walnuts with maple syrup, ground cinnamon, ground nutmeg, and sea salt until evenly coated.
- Transfer the nut mixture onto a parchment paper-lined baking sheet.
- Bake for 10 to 12 minutes, or until the nuts are aromatic and brown, in a preheated oven.
- Before serving, let the walnuts and spiced maple pecans cool.

Nutritional Value:

- Calories: 220 kcal
- Protein: 4g

Copyrighted Material

- Fat: 20g
- Carbohydrates: 8g
- Fiber: 3g
- Sugar: 3g

Honey-Roasted Almond Crunch

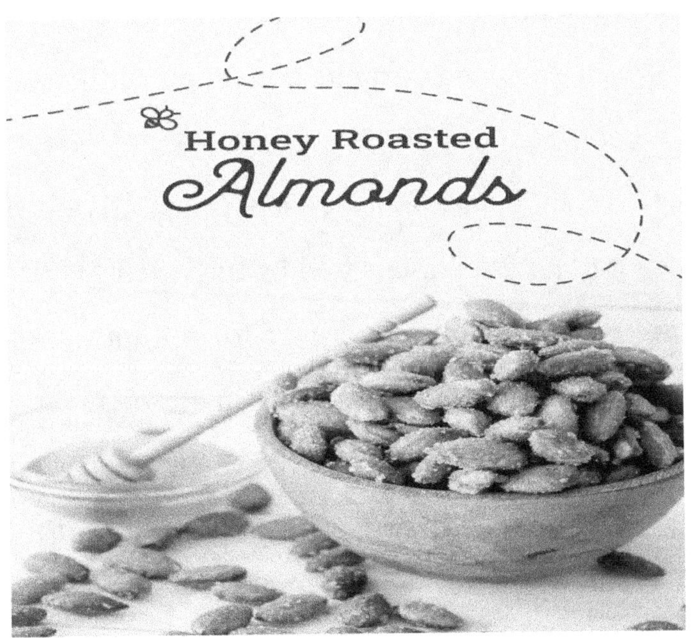

Ingredients:

- 1 cup whole almonds
- 1 tablespoon honey

Copyrighted Material

- 1/2 teaspoon vanilla extract

- 1/4 teaspoon sea salt

- 1/8 teaspoon ground cinnamon

Preparation:

- Preheat the oven to 325°F (163°C).

- Mix almonds with honey, vanilla extract, sea salt, and ground cinnamon until well coated.

- Arrange the honey-roasted almonds on a parchment paper-lined baking sheet.

- Bake the almonds for 15 to 18 minutes, or until they are caramelized and brown.

- Let the almonds that have been roasted with honey to completely cool before serving.

Nutritional Value:

- Calories: 200 kcal

- Protein: 6g

Copyrighted Material

- Fat: 15g

- Carbohydrates: 15g

- Fiber: 3g

- Sugar: 9g

Chili-Lime Cashew Medley

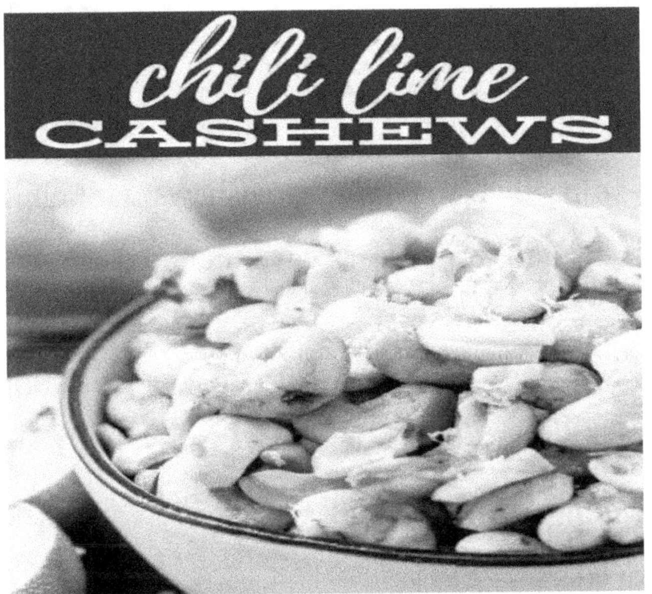

Ingredients:

- 1 cup cashews

- 1 tablespoon olive oil

- 1 teaspoon chili powder

Copyrighted Material

- 1/2 teaspoon lime zest
- 1/4 teaspoon cayenne pepper
- 1/4 teaspoon sea salt

Preparation:

- Heat the olive oil in a pan over medium heat.
- Add cashews and sauté for 2-3 minutes until they begin to turn golden.
- In a bowl mix sautéed cashews with chili powder, lime zest, cayenne pepper, and sea salt until evenly coated.
- Allow the chili-lime cashews to cool before serving.

Nutritional Value:

- Calories: 230 kcal
- Protein: 6g
- Fat: 18g
- Carbohydrates: 13g

Copyrighted Material

- Fiber: 2g
- Sugar: 2g

Enjoy these nourishing nut mixes as a flavorful and wholesome snack. Perfect for satisfying your cravings while providing a dose of healthy fats and nutrients.

Tasty Veggie Bites

Zesty Avocado Cucumber Rolls

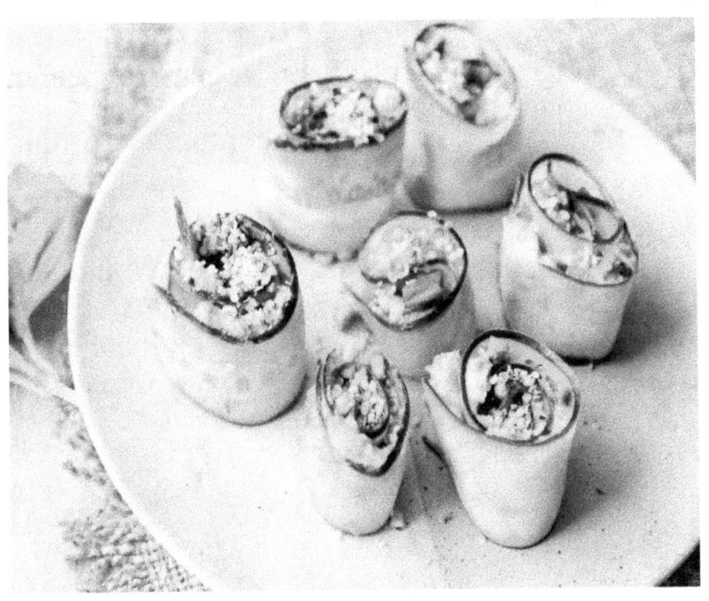

Copyrighted Material

Ingredients:

- 1 large cucumber
- 1 ripe avocado
- 1 tablespoon fresh lime juice
- 1/4 cup cherry tomatoes, diced
- 2 tablespoons red onion, finely chopped
- 1 tablespoon fresh cilantro, chopped
- Salt and pepper to taste
- Microgreens for garnish

Preparation:

- Using a mandoline or vegetable peeler, peel and slice the cucumber into thin strips.
- Mash the ripe avocado in a bowl and add salt, pepper, sliced red onion, diced cherry tomatoes, and fresh cilantro.

Copyrighted Material

- Arrange the strips of cucumber and equally coat each one with the avocado mixture.

- If necessary, use toothpicks to secure the cucumber strips as you roll them up.

- Before serving, garnish these tangy avocado cucumber rolls with microgreens.

Nutritional Value:

- Calories: 120 kcal

- Protein: 2g

- Fat: 10g

- Carbohydrates: 8g

- Fiber: 4g

- Sugar: 2g

Copyrighted Material

Spinach and Feta Stuffed Mushrooms

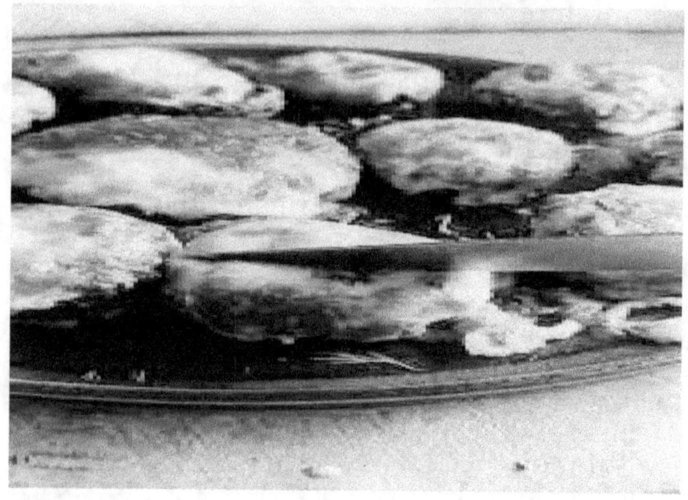

Ingredients:

- 12 large mushrooms, cleaned and stems removed
- 1 cup fresh spinach, chopped
- 1/2 cup feta cheese, crumbled
- 2 tablespoons olive oil
- 2 cloves garlic, minced
- Salt and pepper to taste
- Fresh parsley for garnish

Copyrighted Material

Preparation:

- Set oven temperature to 375°F, or 190°C.

- In a pan over medium heat, warm up the olive oil. Once the garlic is minced, sauté it until flavorful.

- Add the chopped spinach to the pan and let it cook completely.

- Combine the crumbled feta cheese, salt, and pepper with the sautéed spinach in a bowl.

- Insert the feta and spinach mixture into each mushroom cap.

- Spread the packed mushrooms out on a baking sheet and bake for 15 to 18 minutes in a preheated oven.

- Add some fresh parsley as a garnish before serving these delicious feta and spinach filled mushrooms.

Copyrighted Material

Nutritional Value:

- Calories: 90 kcal
- Protein: 4g
- Fat: 7g
- Carbohydrates: 5g
- Fiber: 2g
- Sugar: 2g

Baked Buffalo Cauliflower Bites

Copyrighted Material

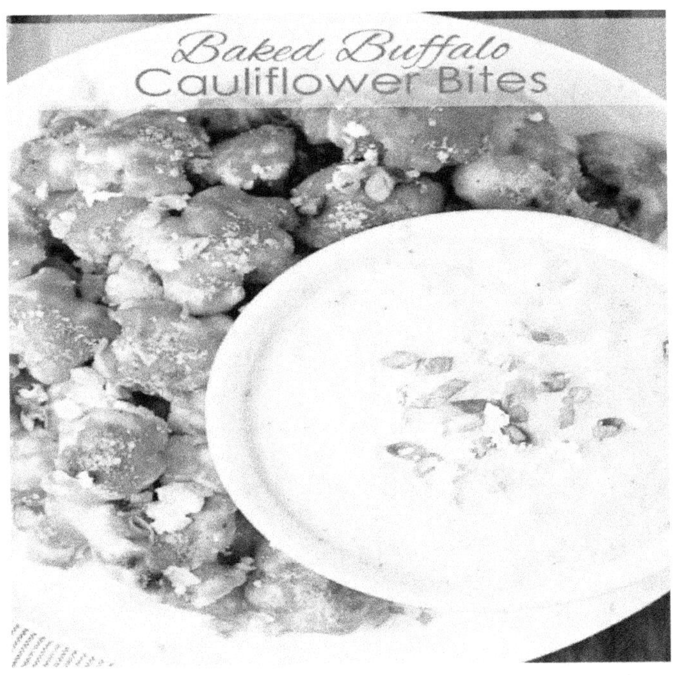

Ingredients:

- 1 cauliflower head, cut into florets
- 1/2 cup buffalo sauce
- 2 tablespoons melted butter
- 1 teaspoon garlic powder
- 1/2 teaspoon onion powder
- 1/4 teaspoon smoked paprika
- Ranch dressing for dipping

Preparation:

- Preheat your oven to 450°F (232°C).
- In a mixing bowl, combine the buffalo sauce, melted butter, garlic powder, onion powder, and smoked paprika.
- Toss the cauliflower florets with the buffalo sauce mixture until well covered.
- Place the coated cauliflower on a baking sheet covered with parchment paper.
- Bake in a preheated oven for 20-25 minutes, or until the cauliflower is crisp.
- For an extra flavor boost, top these baked buffalo cauliflower bits with ranch dressing.

Nutritional Value:

- Calories: 120 kcal
- Protein: 3g
- Fat: 8g

Copyrighted Material

- Carbohydrates: 10g
- Fiber: 4g
- Sugar: 3g

These tasty veggie bites offer a variety of flavors and textures, making them perfect for snacking or serving as appetizers for gatherings. Enjoy the freshness and creativity of these vegetable-based bites.

Copyrighted Material

CHAPTER 7: SWEET TREATS

Guilt-Free Dessert Delights

Dark Chocolate-Dipped Strawberries

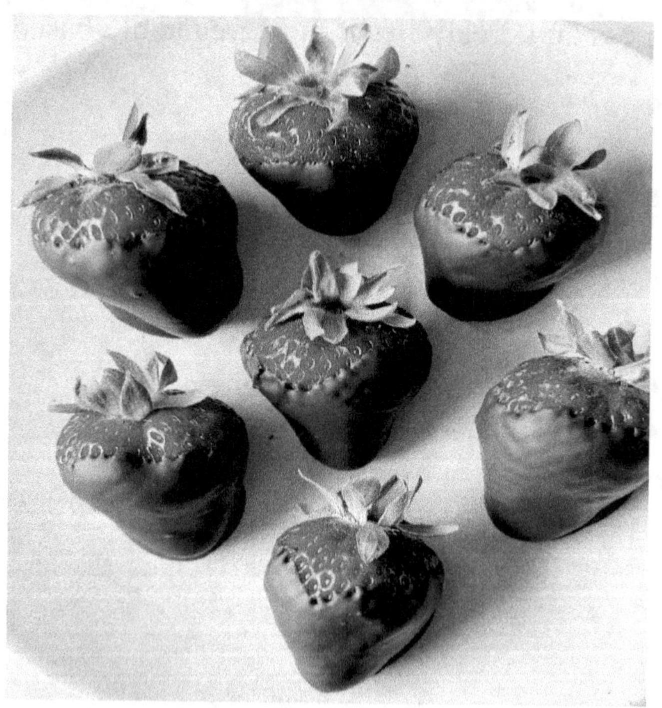

Ingredients:

- 1 cup dark chocolate chips

Copyrighted Material

- 1 pint of fresh, dried and cleaned strawberries

Preparation:

- In a microwave-safe dish, melt dark chocolate chips in 20-second intervals, stirring between each one, until smooth.

- Hold each strawberry by its green stem, put it halfway into the melted dark chocolate.

- Place the coated strawberries on a parchment-lined dish.

- Refrigerate for 15 minutes to set the chocolate.

- Enjoy these guilt-free dark chocolate-dipped strawberries!

Nutritional Value:

- Calories: 60 kcal (per strawberry)
- Protein: 1g

Copyrighted Material

- Fat: 4g

- Carbohydrates: 8g

- Fiber: 2g

- Sugar: 5g

Greek Yogurt Parfait with Fresh Berries

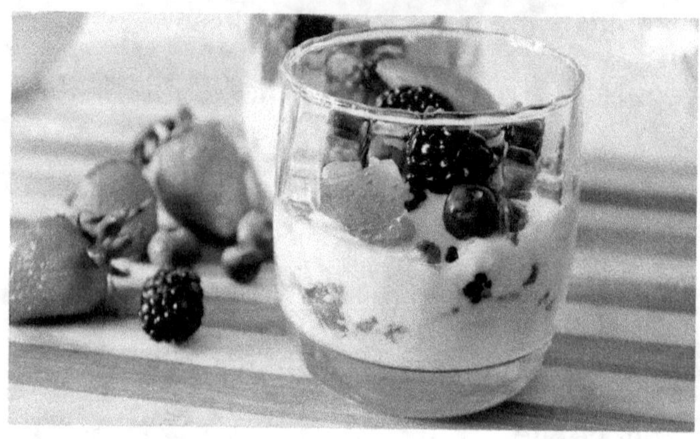

Ingredients:

- cup plain Greek yogurt

- 1 tablespoon honey

- 1/2 cup mixed berries (blueberries, raspberries, strawberries)

- 1 tablespoon slivered almonds

Copyrighted Material

Preparation:

- Layer plain Greek yogurt with mixed berries in a glass or bowl.

- Drizzle honey over the yogurt and berries.

- Sprinkle slivered almonds on top for added crunch.

- Enjoy this guilt-free Greek yogurt parfait as a satisfying dessert.

Nutritional Value:

- Calories: 220 kcal

- Protein: 18g

- Fat: 10g

- Carbohydrates: 20g

- Fiber: 4g

- Sugar: 14g

Copyrighted Material

Banana-Oat Blender Muffins

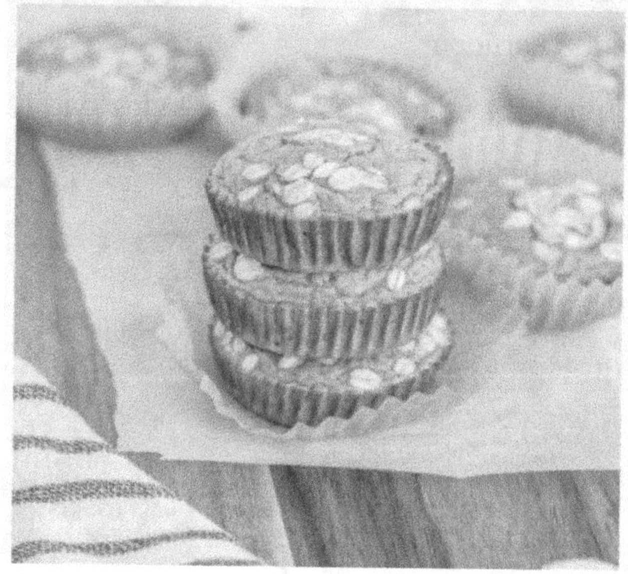

Ingredients:

- 2 ripe bananas
- 2 cups rolled oats
- 2 large eggs
- 1 cup plain Greek yogurt

Copyrighted Material

- 1/4 cup honey

- 1 teaspoon vanilla extract

- 1 teaspoon baking powder

- 1/2 teaspoon baking soda

- 1/4 teaspoon salt

- Dark chocolate chips (optional)

Preparation:

- Preheat the oven to 350°F (175°C) and line a muffin tin with paper liners.

- Blend ripe bananas, rolled oats, eggs, Greek yogurt, honey, vanilla extract, baking powder, baking soda, and salt until smooth.

- Pour batter into muffin tin, filling each cup two-thirds full.

- Optional: Sprinkle a few dark chocolate chips on top of each muffin.

- Bake for 18-20 minutes, or until a toothpick inserted in the center comes out clean.
- Cool before enjoying these guilt-free banana-oat blender muffins.

Nutritional Value:

- Calories: 150 kcal (per muffin)
- Protein: 6g
- Fat: 4g
- Carbohydrates: 25g
- Fiber: 3g
- Sugar: 8g

These guilt-free desserts provide a sweet and satisfying end to your meal without compromising on health. Enjoy the natural sweetness of fresh fruits, yogurt, and wholesome ingredients in these delicious treats.

Copyrighted Material

Indulgent Yet Healthy Sweets

Chocolate Avocado Mousse

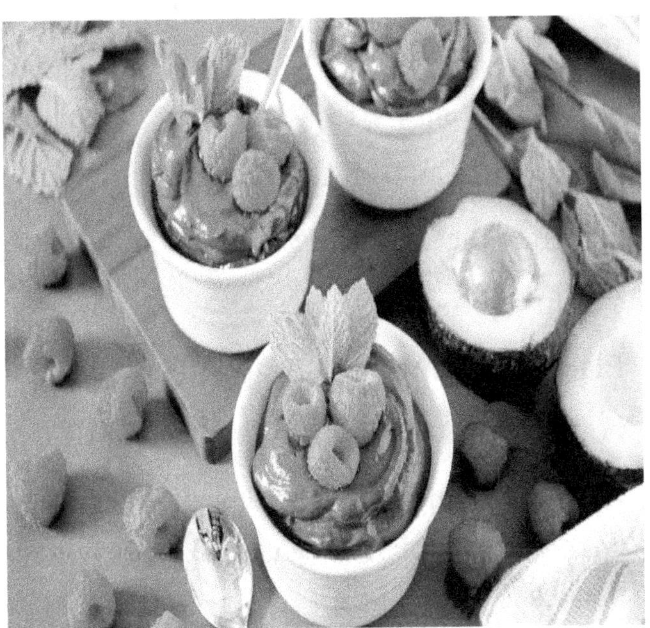

Ingredients:

- 2 ripe avocados

- 1/2 cup unsweetened cocoa powder

- 1/4 cup honey or maple syrup

- 1 teaspoon vanilla extract

- Pinch of salt

- Fresh berries for garnish

Copyrighted Material

Preparation:

- In a food processor or blender, mix the ripe avocados, cocoa powder, honey or maple syrup, vanilla essence, and a sprinkle of salt.

- Blend until smooth and creamy.

- Transfer the chocolate avocado mousse to serving glasses.

- Place in the refrigerator for at least half an hour, before serving.

- Before serving this luscious and nutritious chocolate mousse, garnish with fresh berries.

Nutritional Value:

- Calories: 200 kcal (per serving)

- Protein: 4g

- Fat: 15g

- Carbohydrates: 20g

- Fiber: 7g

- Sugar: 9g

Copyrighted Material

Nutty Banana Bread Bites

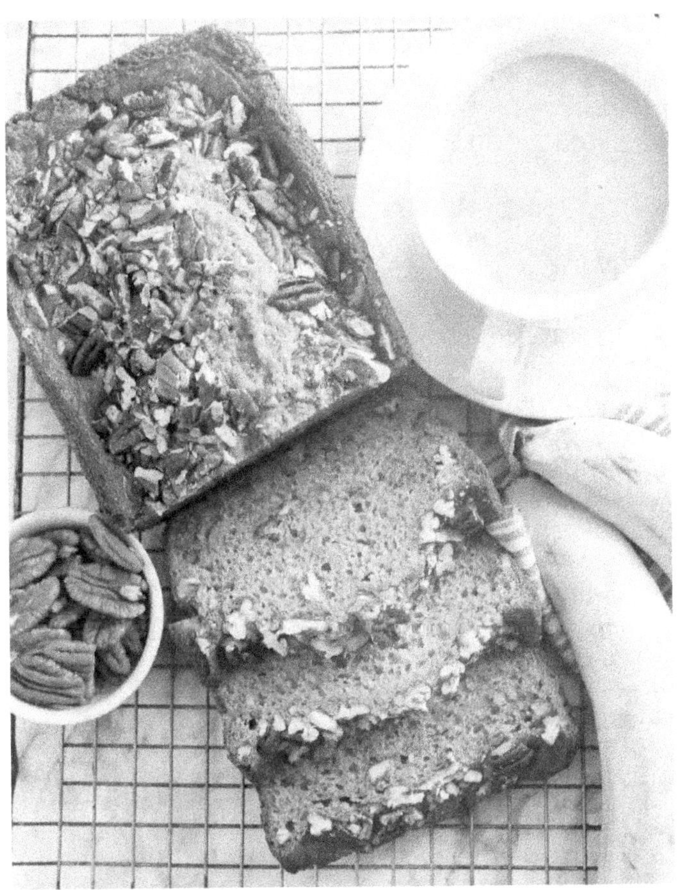

Ingredients:

- 2 ripe bananas, mashed
- 1 cup almond flour

Copyrighted Material

- 1/4 cup coconut flour
- 1/4 cup almond butter
- 1/4 cup honey or maple syrup
- 1 teaspoon vanilla extract
- 1/2 teaspoon baking soda
- 1/4 teaspoon cinnamon
- Pinch of salt
- Chopped nuts (walnuts or pecans) for topping

Preparation:

- Preheat your oven to 350°F (175°C) and prepare a baking pan by lining it with parchment paper.
- In a bowl mix mashed bananas, almond flour, coconut flour, almond butter, honey or maple syrup, vanilla extract, baking soda, cinnamon, and a pinch of salt. Until well combined.

Copyrighted Material

- Scoop spoonfuls of batter onto the prepared baking pan, forming bite-sized cookies.
- Top each cookie with chopped nuts.
- Bake for 12-15 minutes until the edges are golden.
- Cool before serving these nutty banana bread bites.

Nutritional Value:

- Calories: 120 kcal (per bite)
- Protein: 3g
- Fat: 8g
- Carbohydrates: 12g
- Fiber: 2g
- Sugar: 6g

Copyrighted Material

Raspberry Chia Seed Pudding

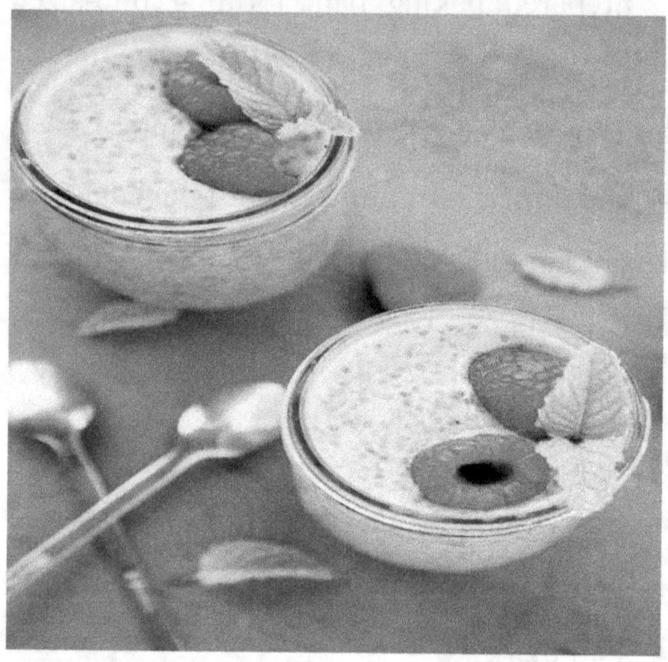

Ingredients:

- 1/2 cup chia seeds
- 2 cups unsweetened almond milk
- 1 tablespoon honey or maple syrup
- 1 teaspoon vanilla extract
- 1 cup fresh raspberries
- Mint leaves for garnish

Copyrighted Material

Preparation:

- Chia seeds, almond milk, honey (or maple syrup), and vanilla essence should all be combined in a bowl.

- To prevent clumps, let the mixture remain for ten minutes before whisking it once again.

- Chia seed pudding should be refrigerated for two hours or overnight.

- Arrange the fresh raspberries on top of the chia seed pudding in serving glasses.

- Before serving this decadent yet healthful raspberry chia seed pudding, garnish with mint leaves.

Nutritional Value:

- Calories: 180 kcal (per serving)
- Protein: 5g
- Fat: 9g

Copyrighted Material

- Carbohydrates: 20g
- Fiber: 10g
- Sugar: 6g

These indulgent yet healthy sweet treats offer a balance of rich flavors and wholesome ingredients. Enjoy the satisfaction of dessert without compromising on your health goals.

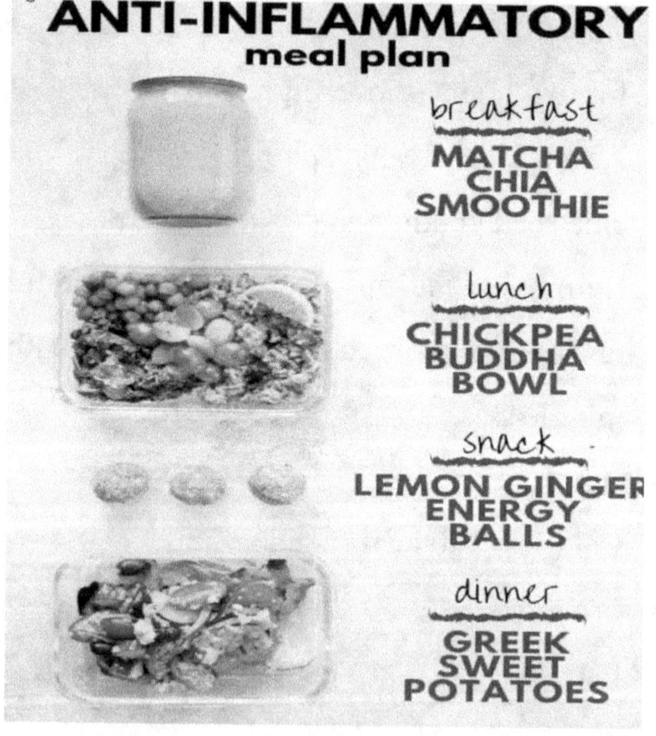

Copyrighted Material

CHAPTER 8: MASTERING THE ART OF MEAL PREPARATION

Batch Cooking Techniques for Efficiency

Strategic Ingredient Prep:

- Get a head start by washing, peeling, and chopping vegetables in advance.

- Enhance flavor by marinating proteins with preferred seasonings and storing them in portioned containers.

- Simplify the process by pre-measuring dry ingredients like spices, grains, and legumes.

Efficient One-Pot Meals:

- Minimize cleanup by opting for dishes that can be cooked in a single pot or pan.

Copyrighted Material

- Explore the versatility of stews, casseroles, or stir-fries with a variety of ingredients.

Batch Roasting:

- Roast a large batch of vegetables, including sweet potatoes, carrots, and Brussels sprouts.

- Prepare roasted chicken breasts or thighs seasoned with versatile herbs and spices.

Grains and Legumes:

- Cook a surplus of grains such as quinoa, brown rice, or farro for easy meal assembly.

- Have a ready supply of cooked beans or lentils to incorporate into various dishes.

Freezing Portions:

- Streamline future meals by portioning them into freezer-safe containers for convenient thawing and reheating.

Copyrighted Material

- Ensure easy identification by labeling containers with the preparation date and contents.

Multi-Tasking Appliances:

- Maximize efficiency by using slow cookers, Instant Pots, or pressure cookers to simultaneously prepare multiple components.

- Achieve a complete meal by cooking proteins, grains, and vegetables in one appliance.

Weekly Meal Prep Sessions:

- Establish a routine by designating a specific time each week for batch cooking.

- Prevent monotony by planning a diverse menu for the upcoming week.

Copyrighted Material

Reusable Storage Solutions:

- Invest in sustainable storage options such as glass or BPA-free plastic containers for prepared ingredients.
- Opt for silicone bags when freezing soups, stews, or sauces.

Pre-Chopped and Frozen Ingredients:

- Save time by purchasing pre-chopped vegetables or fruits.
- Preserve fresh herbs by freezing them in olive oil for effortless seasoning.

Customizable Base Recipes:

- Create versatile base recipes that can be transformed into various meals.
- For instance, a tomato-based sauce can serve as a base for pasta, pizza, or soup.

Copyrighted Material

Smart Organization:

- Optimize efficiency by arranging ingredients in the order of use during cooking.
- Maintain a well-organized pantry with essential staples for quick access.

Themed Cuisine Days:

- Introduce variety by assigning specific days for themed cuisines, allowing for bulk preparation of similar ingredients.
- For example, a Mexican-themed day can include preparing rice, beans, and seasoned meats.

Mindful Portioning:

- Prevent overcooking by portioning meals according to serving sizes.
- For accurate measures, use a kitchen scale.

Copyrighted Material

Labeling and Dating:

- Ensure freshness and timely consumption by clearly labeling containers with preparation dates and contents.
- Adopt a rotation system, placing older items at the front for prioritized use.

Adaptable Sauces and Dressings:

- Elevate flavors by creating versatile sauces and dressings that complement a range of dishes.
- Store these in separate containers for convenient drizzling over meals.

Efficient batch cooking not only saves time but also guarantees a diverse array of nutritious meals throughout the week. Tailor these techniques to suit individual preferences and dietary needs.

Copyrighted Material

Planning and Organizing Your Weekly Anti-Inflammatory Meals

Menu Planning:

- Craft a weekly menu incorporating diverse anti-inflammatory foods.
- Ensure a balance of proteins, grains, veggies, and fruits.

Ingredient Checklist:

- Simplify your shopping by creating a comprehensive list based on your planned menu.
- Check your pantry to avoid unnecessary duplicate purchases.

Seasonal Selections:

- Prioritize freshness and optimal nutritional value by choosing seasonal fruits and vegetables.

Copyrighted Material

- Experiment with different seasonal produce to add variety to your meals.

Protein Variety:

- Achieve a balanced diet by including lean proteins like fish, poultry, legumes, and plant-based options.

- Rotate protein sources throughout the week for a well-rounded nutritional intake.

Grain Diversity:

- Boost nutritional benefits by incorporating a variety of whole grains such as quinoa, brown rice, oats, and barley.

- Experiment with ancient grains to diversify your nutrient intake.

Colorful Plate:

- Aim for a vibrant plate filled with a mix of colorful fruits and vegetables.

Copyrighted Material

- Different colors often signify diverse antioxidants and phytonutrients.

Batch Cooking Sessions:

- Save time during the week by dedicating specific days for batch cooking.

- Prepare staples like grains, proteins, and sauces in advance for quick and easy meals.

Balanced Nutrients:

- Ensure a balanced intake of macronutrients, including proteins, fats, and carbohydrates, in each meal.

- Incorporate healthy fats from sources like avocados, olive oil, and nuts.

Hydration Strategy:

- Plan your daily water intake and add variety with herbal teas or infused water.

- Stay hydrated to support overall well-being and reduce inflammation.

Copyrighted Material

Mindful Snacking:

- Plan nutritious snacks, such as fresh fruit, vegetable sticks with hummus, or a handful of nuts.
- Avoid processed snacks high in sugars and unhealthy fats.

Adaptable Recipes:

- Choose recipes that allow for ingredient substitutions based on availability.
- Be flexible in adapting recipes to suit your taste and dietary needs.

Portion Control:

- Practice mindful eating and portion control to avoid overeating.
- Use smaller plates to create a visual cue for portion sizes.

Copyrighted Material

Prep-ahead Breakfasts:

- Start your day right with grab-and-go options like overnight oats, chia seed pudding, or smoothie packs.
- Ensure a nutritious breakfast without compromising time.

Refrigerator Organization:

- Keep your refrigerator organized with labeled containers for easy access.
- Ensure perishable items are visible to prevent waste.

Flexible Planning:

- Be flexible in your meal plan to adjust for unexpected events.
- Have backup options for busy days or when dining out.

Organizing your weekly anti-inflammatory meals involves thoughtful planning and a

Copyrighted Material

commitment to a diverse and nutrient-rich diet. By incorporating these strategies, you can create a well-balanced and delicious weekly menu that supports your health goals.

Tips for Storage, Preservation, and Reheating

Smart Storage Tips:

Airtight Containers:

- Keep your meals fresh in airtight containers to preserve flavors and prevent unwanted odors.

Labeling and Dating:

- Stay organized by dating and labeling containers in your fridge or freezer.
- Prioritize older items first with a simple rotation system.

Copyrighted Material

Freezer-Friendly Packaging:

- Invest in freezer-safe bags or containers for extended storage periods.

- Avoid freezer burn by removing excess air from freezer bags.

Portion Control:

- Simplify your reheating process by dividing meals into individual portions.

- This way, you only thaw what you need, minimizing waste.

Use Glass Containers:

- Opt for glass containers over plastic for storage, as they are more resistant to odors and stains.

- Glass is also microwave-safe for easy reheating.

Copyrighted Material

Preservation Techniques:

Vacuum Sealing:

- Extend the freshness of your foods by vacuum-sealing them, reducing the risk of freezer burn.

Herb Infused Oils:

- Preserve herbs in olive oil to add flavor to your dishes.

- Use ice cube trays for portioning and freezing these herb-infused oils.

Blanching Vegetables:

- Maintain the color, flavor, and nutrition of vegetables by blanching before freezing.

- Shock them in ice water and pat dry before freezing.

Citrus Preservation:

- Preserve citrus fruits by zesting and juicing, then freezing in ice cube trays.

Copyrighted Material

- These cubes can be added to recipes for a burst of flavor.

Homemade Sauces:

- Make and store homemade sauces in small batches.
- Freeze in portions to enhance the flavor of future meals.

Effective Reheating Tips:

Microwave Smartly:

- Reheat meals in the microwave using short intervals, stirring between each interval.
- Arrange food evenly on the plate for consistent reheating.

Oven Reheating:

- Retain moisture in baked dishes by reheating them at a low temperature and covering them with foil.

Copyrighted Material

Stovetop Reheating:

- Use a non-stick skillet or saucepan for stovetop reheating.

- Pour in a little water or broth to prevent it from sticking.

Thawing Safely:

- Achieve even thawing by placing frozen meals in the refrigerator overnight.

- Use the microwave's defrost setting as an alternative.

Check Internal Temperature:

- When reheating proteins, ensure they reach a safe internal temperature to avoid foodborne illnesses.

- Use a food thermometer to check temperatures.

Copyrighted Material

Bonus Tips for Smart Kitchen Management:

Plan Rotation:

- Minimize waste and keep things fresh by regularly rotating items in your freezer and refrigerator.

Monitor Expiry Dates:

- Safeguard against spoilage by paying attention to expiration dates, especially for frozen items.
- Discard any items that show signs of freezer burn or spoilage.

Season After Reheating:

- Add a final touch of freshness by incorporating fresh herbs, spices, or a squeeze of citrus after reheating.
- This maintains the vibrancy of the dish.

By adopting these clever tips, you'll effortlessly master the art of food storage, preservation, and

Copyrighted Material

reheating, ensuring your anti-inflammatory meals remain both delicious and nutritious throughout the week.

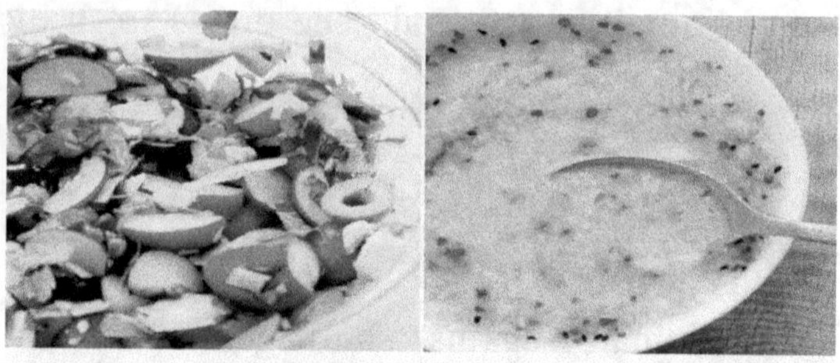

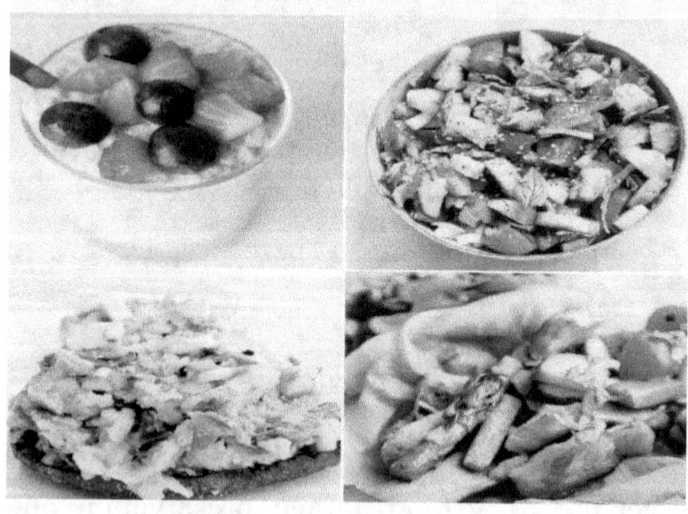

Copyrighted Material

CHAPTER 9: TIPS FOR DINING OUT

Making Healthy Choices

Don't let dining out hinder your commitment to healthy eating! Here are practical tips to guide you in making smart choices while relishing delicious meals without compromising your anti-inflammatory goals:

Before Your Outing:

- **Conduct Research:** Review online menus in advance, pinpointing restaurants offering anti-inflammatory options like lean proteins, vibrant vegetables, and whole grains.

- **Meal Planning:** Decide your order beforehand to sidestep impromptu choices influenced by hunger or temptation.

Copyrighted Material

- **Healthy Snacks:** Bring along small, nutritious snacks like a salad, nuts, seeds, or yogurt to deter overindulgence in unhealthy appetizers.

Ordering Strategies:

- **Protein and Fiber Focus:** Opt for lean proteins such as grilled chicken, fish, or tofu. Pair them with fiber-rich sides like roasted vegetables, quinoa, or brown rice.

- **Embrace Greens:** Load your plate with colorful vegetables, favoring steamed or roasted options over fried or cream-based alternatives.

- **Moderate Extras:** Avoid heavily sauced or cheesy dishes. Request dressings and sauces on the side to control consumption.

- **Share the Load:** Considering generous restaurant portions, share a meal with a friend to control your intake.

Copyrighted Material

Mindful Eating:

- **Enjoy Every Bite:** Slow down, savor the flavors, and chew deliberately to sense fullness faster, preventing overeating.

- **Pay Attention to Your Body:** Don't overeat; instead, stop when you're satisfied. Avoid the need to finish everything on your plate.

- **Stay Hydrated:** Drink water throughout the meal to curb hunger and differentiate thirst from hunger.

Bonus Tips:

- **Inquire About Ingredients:** Ask your server about ingredients and cooking methods. Choose dishes prepared with healthy oils and minimal added sugar.

- **Be Assertive:** Don't hesitate to request modifications, like grilled instead of fried

Copyrighted Material

options or omitting cheese and unhealthy toppings.

- **Plan Ahead:** If you do indulge in something unhealthy, plan a healthier meal for your next outing or at home to help balance things out.

Dining out can be enjoyable while aligning with an anti-inflammatory lifestyle. By implementing these tips and making informed choices, relish your restaurant experience while staying on track with your health goals. So, gather your friends, head to your favorite spot, and delight in flavors without compromising your well-being!

Navigating Restaurant Menus

Navigating the mysteries of restaurant menus with an anti-inflammatory focus can be tricky. Master this culinary journey with savvy tactics,

Copyrighted Material

ensuring every meal is a delightful and healthy experience. Here are the tips to guide your choices:

Pre-Restaurant Planning:

- **Research is Key:** Before entering, explore online menus or call ahead to spot potential anti-inflammatory options. Seek terms like "grilled," "baked," "steamed," "whole grain," and "colorful vegetables."

- **Strategic Planning:** Decide on your main dish and sides in advance, avoiding impulsive choices driven by hunger or enticing descriptions.

- **Smart Backup:** Bring a small, nutritious snack like nuts, seeds, or fruit to resist unhealthy appetizers or bread baskets.

Copyrighted Material

Menu Decoding:

- **Protein Powerhouse Hunt:** Prioritize lean proteins like grilled chicken, fish, or tofu, avoiding heavily breaded or battered options.

- **Veggie Vanguard**: Embrace the power of colorful vegetables! Opt for steamed, roasted, or grilled choices, steering clear of fried or cream-laden temptations. Aim for at least half your plate to be veggies.

- **Fiber Friends:** Choose fiber-rich sides like quinoa, brown rice, roasted sweet potato, or steamed broccoli for lasting satisfaction.

- **Sauce Scrutiny:** Beware of sauces and dressings loaded with hidden sugars or unhealthy fats. Request them on the side, opting for lighter choices like olive oil and vinegar.

Copyrighted Material

- **Wordplay Wisdom:** Exercise caution with menu terms like "crispy," "creamy," "rich," or "fried" – often signaling less-healthy cooking methods and added fats.

Ordering with Confidence:

- **Don't Be Shy:** Your server is there to help. Inquire about ingredients, cooking methods, and portion sizes.

- **Modification Mastery:** Customize your order fearlessly. Opt for grilled or baked instead of fried, request sauces on the side, or omit cheese and unhealthy toppings.

- **Share the Joy:** Consider splitting a meal with a friend to control your intake and potentially save money.

Copyrighted Material

Bonus Tips:

- **Hydration Hero:** Sip water throughout your meal for satiety and to prevent overeating.

- **Mindful Munching:** Savor each bite, and chew deliberately, aiding digestion and preventing overindulgence.

- **Body Listening:** Stop eating when satisfied, not overly full. Resist finishing everything on your plate.

- **Next Time's Plan:** If indulging in something less healthy, plan a more anti-inflammatory meal for your next outing or at home for balance.

Remember, navigating restaurant menus with an anti-inflammatory focus is a journey, not a destination. Be patient, experiment, and find what works for you. With savvy choices, you can conquer the culinary world, relishing

Copyrighted Material

delicious, healthy meals that support your well-being!

Socializing and Celebrating While Staying True to Your Goals

Socializing and celebrating are life's essentials, and balancing health goals during gatherings is an art. Fear not! Navigate social events while staying true to your anti-inflammatory principles with these tips:

Before the Gathering:

- **Smart Fueling:** Eat a healthy meal beforehand to avoid arriving famished and making impulsive choices.

- **Hydration Focus:** Stay energized by drinking water throughout the day and during the event.

- **Pack a Backup:** Carry healthy snacks like nuts, seeds, or fruit if options are limited.
- **Strategic Planning:** Pre-strategize healthier alternatives if unhealthy options dominate.

Navigating the Menu:

- **Appetizer Agility:** Opt for lighter choices like veggie crudités, hummus with whole-wheat pita, or grilled skewers. Skip fried treats and heavy dips.
- **Main Course Maneuvers:** Seek lean proteins paired with veggies or whole grains. Avoid creamy sauces and heavy breading.
- **Salad Savvy:** Choose salads with greens and colorful veggies, opting for a light vinaigrette on the side.

Copyrighted Material

- **Wise Sips:** Stick to water, unsweetened iced tea, or sparkling water with a lime wedge. Limit sugary cocktails and sodas.

Party Strategies:

- **Contributor Role:** Offer a healthy appetizer or side dish to share, ensuring at least one option aligns with your goals.

- **Personal Beverage:** Carry a reusable water bottle or infused water for a refreshing and healthy drink.

- **Social Engagement:** Focus on conversations and mingling rather than fixating on food.

- **Mindful Munching:** Savor bites and listens to your body's hunger cues, avoiding mindless snacking.

- **Portion Control:** Use smaller plates to manage intake and prevent overindulging.

Copyrighted Material

Celebration Hacks:

- **Dance Delight:** Celebrate through dance! It's a fun way to burn calories and enjoy life without relying on food.

- **Interactive Fun:** Suggest games or activities to shift the focus from food to connecting with others.

- **Joyful Moments:** Remember, celebrations are about cherished moments with loved ones. Create memories beyond the table.

Bonus Tips:

- **Moderation Mindset:** It's okay to enjoy treats in moderation. Savor mindfully.

- **Honesty Matters:** If struggling, explain your dietary choices politely. Most people will be understanding and supportive.

Copyrighted Material

- **Practice makes Progress:** Improving your ability to navigate social situations with food challenges is a gradual process. The more you engage in it, the more comfortable and adept you become over time.

Celebrating and maintaining your health go hand-in-hand. With planning, mindful choices, and a focus on connection, you can enjoy social events without compromising your anti-inflammatory journey. Raise a glass of water, embrace joy, and savor the celebration, knowing you are making choices that prioritize your well-being!

Copyrighted Material

CHAPTER 10: LIFESTYLE TIPS FOR LONG-TERM SUCCESS

Incorporating Exercise

Absolutely! Exercise stands out as a formidable ally in your anti-inflammatory journey, boosting your overall well-being in numerous ways:

Physical Benefits:

- **Inflammation Control:** Engaging in regular physical activity serves as a potent regulator, diminishing pro-inflammatory markers and effectively countering chronic inflammation.

- **Optimized Circulation:** Exercise, the catalyst for enhanced blood flow, ensures the efficient delivery of oxygen and vital nutrients to cells and tissues. This not only

Copyrighted Material

reduces inflammation but also accelerates the healing process.

- **Weight Management Mastery:** A consistent exercise regimen contributes significantly to maintaining an optimal weight, directly addressing the risk factors associated with inflammation linked to excess weight.

- **Muscle and Bone Fortitude:** The process of building muscle mass not only aids in burning calories during rest, thereby reducing inflammation but also serves as a protective shield against injuries that could potentially trigger inflammation.

- **Enhanced Sleep Quality:** The positive impact of exercise extends to promoting faster sleep onset and ensuring a more restful sleep, a critical component for overall health and inflammation reduction.

Copyrighted Material

Mental and Emotional Benefits:

- **Reduces stress:** Exercise recognized as a natural stress reliever, exercise actively combats one of the major triggers for inflammation. The release of endorphins during exercise serves as a powerful mood enhancer, effectively reducing anxiety and stress levels.

- **Boosts energy levels:** The ripple effect of regular physical activity manifests in heightened energy levels, empowering individuals to approach each day with increased motivation and vigor.

- **Improves self-esteem:** The journey towards accomplishing fitness milestones isn't just physical—it significantly elevates confidence and self-esteem, fostering a positive outlook and contributing to overall well-being.

Copyrighted Material

Incorporating Exercise

- **Find activities you enjoy:** The key to sustainable exercise habits lies in selecting activities that resonate with personal enjoyment. Whether it's dancing, swimming, cycling, hiking, or team sports, the element of fun ensures greater adherence.

- **Start slow and gradually increase intensity:** Don't try to do too much too soon, especially if you're new to exercise. The gradual progression from short, manageable sessions to extended durations and heightened intensity is a foundational principle. This approach ensures sustainable fitness growth.

- **Variety is key:** Combatting monotony involves integrating a diverse range of exercises—cardio, strength training, and

Copyrighted Material

flexibility workouts. This not only targets various muscle groups but also adds an exciting dimension to the routine.

- **Listen to your body:** The ethos of exercise extends beyond mere activity—listening to your body becomes paramount. Recognizing the need for rest days and refraining from pushing through pain safeguards against potential injuries.

Anti-inflammatory Exercise Tips:

- **Focus on low-impact activities:** Opting for low-impact activities such as swimming, yoga, or walking serves as a protective measure for joints, minimizing stress during exercise.

- **Include anti-inflammatory foods:** Elevate the impact of exercise by synergizing it with a diet rich in

Copyrighted Material

inflammation-fighting foods—fruits, vegetables, whole grains, and healthy fats.

- **Holistic Warm-ups and Cool-downs:** Safeguard against injuries by incorporating meticulous warm-up routines pre-exercise and structured cool-down sessions post-exercise. This practice not only prevents injuries but also expedites the recovery process.

- **Mindful Exercise Dynamics:** Elevating the exercise experience involves a conscious focus on form and breathing. This not only maximizes the benefits derived from each session but also minimizes stress on the body.

Remember, the magic of exercise lies not just in its duration but in its consistency. Commence your journey from your current fitness level, establish a consistent rhythm, and gradually

Copyrighted Material

amplify your activity. With exercise as the cornerstone of your anti-inflammatory lifestyle, a healthier, happier you beckons on the horizon!

Stress Management Techniques

Mindful Breathing:

- Engage in deep, mindful breathing to activate the body's relaxation response.
- Take a deep breath through your nose, hold it, and exhale slowly through your mouth.

Meditation and Mindfulness:

- Foster a calm mind and reduce stress through regular meditation.
- Practice mindfulness techniques, focusing on the present moment for overall well-being.

Copyrighted Material

Yoga for Stress Relief:

- Engage in yoga, which combines physical postures, breath control, and meditation.
- Yoga promotes flexibility, relaxation, and stress reduction.

Progressive Muscle Relaxation (PMR):

- Systematically tense and relax muscle groups with PMR.
- Promote physical relaxation and mental calmness through this technique.

Nature Walks and Outdoor Activities:

- Rejuvenate the mind and minimize stress by connecting with nature.
- Opt for natural escapes like walking, hiking, or gardening.

Journaling and Expressive Writing:

- Reflect on emotions and experiences through a stress journal.

Copyrighted Material

- Use expressive writing to process and release built-up stress.

Digital Detox:

- Disconnect and declutter the mind by taking breaks from electronic devices.
- Establish tech-free zones or times during the day.

Art and Creativity:

- Find therapeutic outlets for stress through creative activities like painting or drawing.
- Engage in artistic expression as a means of relieving stress.

Laughter Therapy:

- Include laughter into your routine through humor, comedy, or socializing.
- Release endorphins and nurture a positive mindset with laughter.

Copyrighted Material

Social Connections:

- Foster strong connections with friends and family.
- Seek support, share experiences, and enjoy the benefits of social interaction.

Massage and Bodywork:

- Alleviate physical tension and foster relaxation with regular massages.
- Treat yourself to bodywork sessions for added stress relief.

Aromatherapy:

- Create a calming environment using essential oils or aromatherapy.
- Explore scents like lavender, chamomile, and eucalyptus for stress relief.

Biofeedback and Relaxation Apps:

- Monitor and manage stress levels with biofeedback tools or relaxation apps.

Copyrighted Material

- Receive real-time feedback on stress responses through these technologies.

Setting Boundaries:

- Protect personal time and space by establishing clear boundaries.
- Prioritize self-care and confidently say "no" when needed for effective stress management.

Gratitude Practice:

- Cultivate a gratitude mindset by acknowledging positive aspects of life.
- Practice gratitude regularly through journaling or verbal affirmations.

Guided Imagery:

- Reduce stress and promote relaxation through guided imagery exercises.
- Visualize serene scenes to create calming mental images.

Copyrighted Material

Professional Support:

- Consult with mental health professionals, counselors, or therapists for guidance and support.
- Access tools and strategies for effective stress management through professional support.

Remember, stress management is a personal journey. Experiment with various methods to create a stress-reduction routine tailored to your preferences and lifestyle.

Sleep Hygiene and Its Impact on Inflammation

Prioritize Consistent Sleep Schedule:

- Stick to a regular sleep-wake cycle by going to bed and waking up at the same time every day.

Copyrighted Material

- Consistency enhances your body's natural rhythm, circadian rhythm, fostering better sleep quality.

Create a Relaxing Bedtime Routine:

- Establish a calming pre-sleep routine with activities like reading or gentle stretching.
- Signal to your body that it's time to wind down for improved relaxation.

Ideal Sleep Environment:

- Create a conducive bedroom setting with a cool, dark, and quiet atmosphere.
- Invest in a comfortable mattress and pillows to enhance sleep quality.

Screen Time Reduction Before Bed:

- Minimize screen exposure at least an hour before bedtime to avoid disruptions.
- Blue light from screens can impact melatonin production, affecting sleep.

Copyrighted Material

Mindful Evening Eating:

- To prevent discomfort and indigestion, steer clear of heavy meals near bedtime.
- Opt for light snacks if necessary, allowing time for digestion before lying down.

Incorporate Daytime Exercise:

- Engage in regular daytime physical activity to promote better sleep.
- Avoid vigorous workouts close to bedtime to prevent sleep interference.

Stress Management:

- Practice stress-reducing activities before bedtime, such as meditation.
- A relaxed state contributes to a more conducive sleep environment.

Strategic Napping:

- Keep daytime naps short (20-30 minutes) and avoid late afternoon.

Copyrighted Material

- Taking long or late-afternoon naps can interfere with your nighttime sleep.

Fluid Intake Timing:

- Minimize liquid intake close to bedtime to reduce disruptions from bathroom visits.

- Stay hydrated, but space out fluids to prevent nighttime awakenings.

Addressing Sleep Disorders:

- Consult a healthcare professional for persistent sleep issues.

- Conditions like sleep apnea or insomnia can contribute to inflammation.

Natural Light Exposure:

- Get sunlight exposure during the day, especially in the morning.

- Sunlight regulates the internal clock, supporting healthy sleep-wake patterns.

Copyrighted Material

Comfortable Sleep Position:

- Find a sleep position that aligns your spine for overall comfort.

- Proper alignment contributes to better sleep quality and reduces discomfort.

Sleep-Inducing Atmosphere:

- Use aromatherapy with calming scents like lavender.

- Creating a peaceful atmosphere signals the body that it's time for rest.

Adjusting Sleep Duration:

- Pay attention to the amount of sleep that leaves you refreshed and alert.

- Aim for 7-9 hours per night, adjusting based on individual needs.

Prioritizing optimal sleep habits is crucial for holistic health, impacting inflammation regulation, immune function, and overall

Copyrighted Material

well-being. Experiment with these practices to discover a personalized sleep routine that aligns with your lifestyle and enhances your sleep quality.

Copyrighted Material

CONCLUSION

Celebrating Your Anti-Inflammatory Lifestyle Journey

Reflect on Personal Achievements:

- Pause to acknowledge the positive changes made in adopting an anti-inflammatory lifestyle.

- Celebrate your personal achievements, recognizing that each small step contributes to overall well-being.

Acknowledge Lifestyle Shifts:

- Recognize the shifts in lifestyle, spanning dietary choices, stress management, and sleep patterns.

- Appreciate the commitment shown in nurturing a healthier and more balanced life.

Copyrighted Material

Embrace the Holistic Approach:

- Embrace the holistic approach taken to address inflammation from comprehensively—nutrition, exercise, stress management, and sleep.

- Understand how these elements collectively contribute to a vibrant and inflammation-free life.

Celebrate Improved Well-Being:

- Celebrate the enhancements in overall well-being, be it increased energy, better mood, or enhanced physical health.

- These positive changes signify the transformative impact of an anti-inflammatory lifestyle.

Express Gratitude for Support:

- Extend gratitude to those who supported you—friends, family, healthcare professionals, or anyone who played a role.

- Recognize their encouragement as a valuable part of your success.

Set New Goals and Intentions:

- Consider setting fresh goals and intentions for ongoing growth.

- Whether refining lifestyle aspects or exploring additional wellness practices, maintain the momentum.

Celebrate Milestones:

- Acknowledge the milestones achieved in adopting an anti-inflammatory lifestyle.

- Each milestone reflects dedication and perseverance.

Share Your Success Story:

- Share your success story to inspire others on their wellness journeys.

Copyrighted Material

- Your experience can motivate positive changes in the lives of those around you.

Revel in Improved Self-Care:

- Revel in enhanced self-care resulting from prioritizing anti-inflammatory practices.

- Recognize that self-care is a continuous journey with daily opportunities for growth.

Celebrate the Present Moment:

- Take a moment to celebrate the present and the progress made.

- Mindfully appreciate the journey, acknowledging that positive changes are an ongoing evolution.

In conclusion, the path to an anti-inflammatory lifestyle is not just a destination but a dynamic journey of self-discovery and well-being. Celebrate the steps taken, express gratitude for

Copyrighted Material

positive changes, and anticipate a future filled with continued growth and vitality.

As you conclude your journey through **"Essential Anti-Inflammatory Recipes for Beginners,"** I extend my heartfelt gratitude. If this book has made even a single positive impact on your path to a healthier lifestyle, your words possess the power to guide and inspire others. Your review isn't merely feedback; it serves as an encouragement to uplift fellow individuals on their path to wellness. Share your insights, spark inspiration, and let your expressions become a force for positive transformation. Together, we can foster a community dedicated to holistic well-being. Thank you for being an integral part of this journey of transformation.

With gratitude,

[PAMELA MONTGOMERY]

Copyrighted Material

APPENDIX

Glossary of Key Terms for Anti-Inflammatory Eating

Inflammation: The body's natural response to injury or infection, often showing redness, swelling, and pain. Chronic inflammation is associated with a range of health issues.

Anti-Inflammatory Foods: Nutrient-rich foods known to reduce inflammation, examples include fruits, vegetables, fatty fish, nuts, and olive oil.

Omega-3 Fatty Acids: Essential fatty acids in fish (like salmon), chia seeds, and flaxseeds. They have anti-inflammatory properties and support heart health.

Polyphenols: Plant compounds with antioxidant properties found in fruits, vegetables, tea, and red wine. They combat oxidative stress and inflammation.

Turmeric: A spice with curcumin, known for anti-inflammatory and antioxidant effects. Commonly used in curry dishes.

Ginger: A root with anti-inflammatory and antioxidant properties, used in cooking or brewed as a tea.

Quercetin: A flavonoid in apples, onions, and berries, known for anti-inflammatory and antioxidant effects.

Probiotics: Beneficial bacteria that support gut health. Found in fermented foods like yogurt, kefir, sauerkraut, and kimchi.

Prebiotics: Non-digestible fibers promoting beneficial gut bacteria, found in garlic, onions, and bananas.

Copyrighted Material

Whole Grains: Grains with bran, germ, and endosperm, providing nutrients and fiber, e.g., brown rice, and quinoa.

Cruciferous Vegetables: Vegetables like broccoli, kale, and Brussels sprouts are rich in antioxidants and anti-inflammatory compounds.

Resveratrol: A compound in red grapes, red wine, and berries, known for anti-inflammatory and heart-protective properties.

Glucosinolates: Sulfur-containing compounds in cruciferous vegetables with potential anti-cancer and anti-inflammatory effects.

Eicosanoids: Signaling molecules in the inflammatory response. Omega-3 fatty acids influence anti-inflammatory eicosanoids.

Lycopene: An antioxidant in tomatoes, watermelon, and pink grapefruit, linked to reduced inflammation.

Copyrighted Material

Capsaicin: The spicy compound in chili peppers, with potential anti-inflammatory and pain-relieving effects.

Fiber: Plant-based carbohydrates promoting digestive health, found in fruits, vegetables, whole grains, and legumes.

Adaptogens: Herbs or substances aiding the body in stress adaptation, e.g., ashwagandha, holy basil.

Hormesis: The idea that exposure to mild stressors, like exercise or certain foods, activates adaptive responses improving resilience and health.

Mediterranean Diet: A diet emphasizing fruits, vegetables, olive oil, fish, and nuts, associated with anti-inflammatory benefits.

Copyrighted Material

Resources for Further Reading

Books:

- **The Anti-Inflammation Cookbook** by Amanda Haas and Dr. Bradly Jacobs

- **"Inflammation Nation:** The First Clinically Proven Eating Plan to End Our Nation's Secret Epidemic" by Floyd H. Chilton is a groundbreaking book that introduces a scientifically validated eating plan to combat the hidden epidemic of inflammation in our society. The author, Floyd H. Chilton, provides evidence-based insights into the crucial role of diet in addressing inflammation, offering readers a proactive approach to enhance their health and well-being.

Copyrighted Material

Websites and Blogs:

- [Harvard Health Blog - Fighting Inflammation with Food] (https://www.health.harvard.edu/blog/fighting-inflammation-with-food-2020050719399)

- [The Inflammation Spectrum] (https://drwillcole.com/books/the-inflammation-spectrum) - Dr. Will Cole's website

Scientific Journals and Articles:

- [Role of Nutrition in Inflammatory Bowel Disease] (https://www.ncbi.nlm.nih.gov/pmc/articles/PMC4579563/) - World Journal of Gastroenterology

- [Anti-inflammatory effects of polyphenols in arthritis] (https://www.ncbi.nlm.nih.gov/pmc/article

Copyrighted Material

s/PMC5872786/) - Journal of Science and Food Agriculture

Podcasts:

- [The Inflammation Spectrum with Dr. Will Cole] (https://drwillcole.com/podcast) - Exploring aspects of inflammation and health

Online Courses:

- [Nutrition, Health, and Lifestyle: Issues and Insights] (https://www.coursera.org/learn/nutrition-health-aging) - Offered by McMaster University on Coursera

Social Media Accounts:

- Follow nutritionists, dietitians, and wellness experts on Instagram and Twitter for updates. Examples: @drmarkhyman, @nutritionschool, @thefoodbabe.

Copyrighted Material

Documentaries:

- Fed Up - Explores the role of processed foods and sugar in inflammation and health.
- The Game Changers - Investigates the impact of plant-based diets on inflammation and athletic performance.

Health Organizations:

- [The World Health Organization (WHO)] (https://www.who.int/) - Resources on global nutrition and health.
- [National Institute of Allergy and Infectious Diseases (NIAID)] (https://www.niaid.nih.gov/) - Information on immune system health.

Apps:

- Download apps for nutrition tracking, mindfulness, and fitness for personalized guidance.

Copyrighted Material

Community Support:

- Join online communities like Reddit's r/anti inflammatory for tips. Remember to consult professionals before lifestyle changes.

These resources offer diverse perspectives for a healthier, anti-inflammatory lifestyle.

www.ingramcontent.com/pod-product-compliance
Lightning Source LLC
Chambersburg PA
CBHW050807260726
48660CB00004B/1293